PELVIC FLOOR DISORDERS

Edited by **Raheela M. Rizvi**

Pelvic Floor Disorders
http://dx.doi.org/10.5772/intechopen.69095
Edited by Raheela M. Rizvi

Contributors

Lynn Stothers, Marwa Mohammed Abdulaziz, Andrew Macnab, Naşide Mangır, Christopher Chapple, Sheila MacNeil, Lubna Razzak, Nidhi Sharma, Sudakshina Chakrabarti, Raheela Mohsin Rizvi

First published in London, United Kingdom, 2018 by IntechOpen
IntechOpen is the global imprint of INTECHOPEN LIMITED, registered in England and Wales, registration number: 11086078, The Shard, 25th floor, 32 London Bridge Street
London, SE19SG – United Kingdom
Printed in Croatia

British Library Cataloguing-in-Publication Data
A catalogue record for this book is available from the British Library

Additional hard copies can be obtained from orders@intechopen.com

Pelvic Floor Disorders, Edited by Raheela M. Rizvi
p. cm.
Print ISBN 978-1-78923-244-8
Online ISBN 978-1-78923-245-5

For EU product safety concerns:
IN TECH d.o.o., Prolaz Marije Krucifikse Kozulić 3, 51000 Rijeka, Croatia,
info@intechopen.com or visit our website at intechopen.com.

Meet the editor

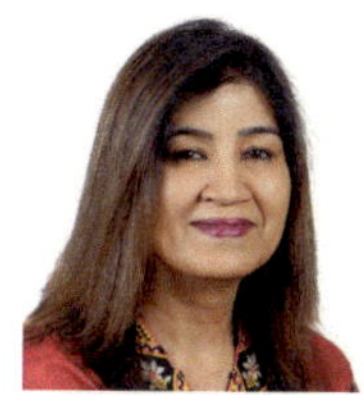

Raheela Mohsin Rizvi is a consultant urogynecologist and has a deep interest in pelvic reconstructive surgery at the Aga Khan University, Karachi, Pakistan. She had her clinical fellowship in urogynecology at the University of Sydney, Australia. Currently, she is a residency program director of Obstetrics and Gynecology and of fellowship in urogynecology and pelvic reconstructive surgery at the Aga Khan University, Pakistan. She has been awarded a certificate of appreciation in recognition of her contribution to the ICS-IUGA Terminology for Female Pelvic Fistulae SSCWG18. She is an editorial board member of five journals and a reviewer of more than 20 indexed journals. She has contributed three chapters related to urogynecology in addition to more than 50 papers in indexed peer-reviewed journals, including the first prevalence study of urinary and fecal incontinence and pelvic organ prolapse in rural Pakistan, which was published in BJOG in 2013.

Contents

Preface

Pelvic floor disorders (PFDs), which include urinary and fecal incontinence (FI) and pelvic organ prolapse (POP), are highly prevalent conditions in women. In the United States alone, this affects almost 25% of women. These disorders often affect women's daily life activities, their sexual function, their ability to exercise, and their social and psychological life. In addition to these, the economic costs for individuals and the society can be astronomical. Conservative management is initially offered, but often enough patients have to be operated upon. In the western countries, for example, 11–21% of women undergo surgery for pelvic organ prolapse, and almost 5–10% of women who have recurrence need a second surgery during their lifetime.

This book *Pelvic Floor Disorders* includes chapters on pathophysiology of pelvic organ prolapse (POP), its treatment by the use of a new synthetic material, treatment for recurrent POP, and diagnostic urogynecology radiology suggesting the use of MRI to diagnose POP considering effects of posture and gravity.

The pathophysiology of pelvic floor disorders (PFDs) is less well understood because it includes both anterior and posterior pelvic compartment disorders. The chapter covers both anatomy and pathophysiology of urinary and fecal incontinence and POP including updates on the subject.

Pelvic organ prolapse is usually a clinical diagnosis. There have been many systems to grade and stage the POP, and yet the diagnosis varies among the experts due to the effects of gravity and posture in which the patients are examined. If it presents with complicated symptoms of posterior compartment defects, then further evaluation is required. MRI is performed in the supine position regardless of the effect of posture and gravity on POP. A full chapter is dedicated to explain in detail the use of a new protocol and advanced technique to evaluate the changes of POP in different positions using open MRI (MRO).

The use of mesh in vaginal surgery for pelvic floor disorders is very debatable. In the last few years, many of the mesh-driven surgical kits have been removed from the market, and surgeons are facing a new challenge to treat recurrent cases of both POP and stress urinary incontinence (SUI). The problems of currently used material polypropylene and designing the ideal material suggested a biodegradable material, poly-L-lactic acid (PLA). The fourth chapter describes a polymer of lactic acid, which is among the most commonly used polymers in biomedical applications.

The last chapter covers the biggest challenge of treating the recurrent cases of POP. Surgical techniques of suspending the vaginal vault with autologous tissue and synthetic mesh are discussed according to clinical presentation and considering the grades of POP. It also includes the role of minimally invasive surgery for recurrent cases.

We have not included the urinary incontinence because there is a separate book published last year. There is a dire need to address fecal incontinence (FI) though we have included posterior compartment defects, but FI has to be included in the upcoming editions.

A word of gratitude is due to the eminent scholars of medical science who contributed the results of their painstaking research for this book.

Raheela M.Rizvi
Obstetrics and Gynecology
Agha Khan University
Karachi, Pakistan

Chapter 1

Introductory Chapter: Pelvic Floor Disorders

Raheela M. Rizvi

Additional information is available at the end of the chapter

http://dx.doi.org/10.5772/intechopen.77302

1. Introduction

The purpose of presenting this book is to provide an insight into various spectrum symptoms that the women present with pelvic floor disorders or/dysfunctions. Pelvic floor disorders and dysfunctions are overlapping terms. Pelvic floor disorders (PFDs) include urinary (UI) and anal incontinence (AI) and pelvic organ prolapse (POP) [1]. To understand pelvic floor dysfunctions, one must appreciate the role of the pelvic floor muscle (PFM). When the PFM is neglected or injured, one or multiple forms of pelvic floor dysfunctions may result, such as bladder and bowel incontinence, obstructive micturition, constipation, pelvic pain and sexual dysfunction, POP and/or low back pain [2].

Pelvic floor dysfunction symptoms of vaginal pain and backache is due to hypertonic pelvic floor muscle which is defined as general increase in muscle tone that can be associated with either elevated contractile activity and/or passive stiffness in the muscle [3]. Most of women present with pelvic floor defects/relaxation symptoms but pelvic floor dysfunction also include non-relaxing pelvic floor symptoms which are not widely recognized. Unlike in pelvic floor disorders caused by relaxed muscles (e.g., pelvic organ prolapse or urinary incontinence, both of which often are identified readily), women affected by no relaxing pelvic floor dysfunction may present with a broad range of nonspecific symptoms. These may include pain and problems with defecation, urination, and sexual function, which require relaxation and coordination of pelvic floor muscles and urinary and anal sphincters. These symptoms may adversely affect the quality of life [4].

2. Etiology, pathophysiology, and risk factors

There are many theories which explain the urinary, fecal incontinence, and pelvic organ prolapse. The risk factors such as obesity, high parity, advanced age, and life style have been

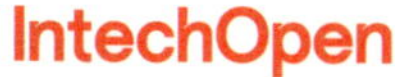

mentioned but we still lack a real understanding of the pathophysiology of pelvic floor disorders. Although it seems apparent that multiple factors combine in each woman for the development of a clinical condition like prolapse or UI, these need to be identified prior to treatment to avoid recurrence of disease. The genetic predisposition aggravated by acquired risk factors, such as childbirth, hormonal changes, and aging predisposes the women to PFD. There is a lack of strong evidence for this hypothesis. Findings of epidemiologic studies are frequently inconsistent. A clearer comprehension of the pathophysiology responsible for PFD is clinically relevant on different levels. First, identifying the patient population at risk through screening of known polymorphism can lead to preventive strategies and the avoidance of contributing risk factors. Second, it may allow the development of interventional therapies where we can locally modify the extracellular matrix (ECM) composition of pelvic floor muscles and ligaments. Future research should then focus on understanding what processes control ECM remodeling and aging using specific and standardized measurement methods and tracing them back to genetic transcription [5].

3. Clinical symptoms and diagnosis

The pelvic floor disorders present with varied symptoms which are related to UI, FI, and POP. Although the women may present with clinical symptom of POP but they usually have backache, vaginal discharge in association with both urinary frequency and urgency and urinary leak while straining or during sexual intercourse. The fecal symptoms may occur after iatrogenic injury to anal sphincters during child birth. The prevalence of pelvic floor dysfunction is 24%, with 16% of women experiencing urinary incontinence, 9% experiencing fecal incontinence, and 3% experiencing pelvic organ prolapse [6]. The clinical presentation of pelvic floor disorders in an urogynecology clinic often lead to a diagnosis where a multidisciplinary approach is usually required for management of a case, which may include evaluation by an urogynecology radiologist. Complete diagnosis by clinical examination alone can be challenging, particularly in cases of posterior vaginal wall prolapse and/or a multicompartment problem. Imaging has become an important complementary tool in the assessment of pelvic floor disorders, and dynamic pelvic floor magnetic resonance imaging (MRI), or MR defecography, has evolved as one of the essential imaging techniques [7].

MRI can simultaneously noninvasively evaluate all pelvic floor compartments and provide information about muscles and ligaments with great contrast resolution, without the use of ionizing radiation and with minimal patient discomfort [8].

4. Treatment

Since pelvic floor disorders present with site-specific defects, clinical presentation varies with grades of disease. The management really depends on the impact of disease on women's quality of life. The first line of management is always conservative which includes pelvic floor muscle physiotherapy, avoidance of risk factors like constipation and smoking but usually women do

http://dx.doi.org/10.5772/intechopen.77302

require a definitive surgical treatment and few women may need a second procedure during their life time. Multi-compartment pelvic floor disorders are now increasingly being evaluated and managed jointly by urogynaecologists and colorectal surgeons in a designated pelvic floor clinic. Before embarking treatment, a comprehensive tool for symptom assessment or the use of a standard questionnaire is required. Patient should be counseled in detail about diagnosis, treatment options, success rate, and complications of a selected procedure.

Author details

Raheela M. Rizvi

Address all correspondence to: raheela.mohsin@aku.edu

Obstetrics and Gynecology, Agha Khan University, Karachi, Pakistan

References

[1] Rogers RG, Pauls RN, Thakar R, et al. An International Urogynecological Association (IUGA)/International Continence Society (ICS) joint report on the terminology for the assessment of sexual health of women with pelvic floor dysfunction. International Urogynecology Journal. 2017 Dec 18;**26**(7):991-996

[2] Unger CA, Weinstein MM, Pretorius DH. Pelvic floor imaging. Obstetrics and Gynecology Clinics of North America. 2011;**38**:23-43

[3] Voorham-van der Zalm PJ, Nijeholt GA LA, Elzevier HW, Putter H, Pelger RC. "Diagnostic investigation of the pelvic floor": A helpful tool in the approach in patients with complaints of micturition, defecation, and/or sexual dysfunction. The Journal of Sexual Medicine. 2008;**5**:864-871

[4] Faubion SS, Shuster LT, Bharucha AE. Recognition and management of nonrelaxing pelvic floor dysfunction. Mayo Clinic Proceedings. 2012;**87**(2):187-193

[5] Campeau L, Gorbachinsky I, Badlani GH, Andersson KE. Pelvic floor disorders: Linking genetic risk factors to biochemical changes. BJU International. 2011 Oct 1;**108**(8):1240-1247

[6] Nygaard I, Barber MD, Burgio KL, et al. Prevalence of symptomatic pelvic floor disorders in US women. JAMA. 2008;**300**:1311-1316

[7] Deegan EG, Stothers L, Kavanagh A, Macnab AJ. Quantification of pelvic floor muscle strength in female urinary incontinence: A systematic review and comparison of contemporary methodologies. Neurourology and Urodynamics. Jan 2018;**37**(1):33-45

[8] Kobi M, Flusberg M, Paroder V, Chernyak V. Practical guide to dynamic pelvic floor MRI. Journal of Magnetic Resonance Imaging. 2018 Mar 25

Chapter 2

Pathophysiology of Pelvic Organ Prolapse

Lubna Razzak

Additional information is available at the end of the chapter

http://dx.doi.org/10.5772/intechopen.76629

Abstract

Pelvic organ support is provided by interaction between the pelvic floor muscle, ligaments and its connective tissues. Failure of anatomical support may result in pelvic organ prolapse. Therefore in managing anterior, posterior, or apical compartments prolapse, conceptual understanding of pelvic floor anatomy is essential for the surgeons. To appropriately treat these entities, comprehension of the various theories of the pathophysiology of pelvic organ prolapse is of paramount importance. DeLancey has described vaginal connective tissue support of the pelvis at three levels that has helped us to understand various clinical manifestations of pelvic organ support dysfunction. Pelvic floor disorder is frequently associated with etiological risk factors which include aging, parity, obesity, connective tissue disorder, increased intra-abdominal pressure and hysterectomy. A better understanding of pathophysiology of muscular, collagen, and neuronal components of the pelvic organs and their support would provide an insight of site specific defects and its prevention.

Keywords: prolapse, anatomy, pelvic floor muscles, compartments, collagen, risk factors

1. Introduction

Approximately one-third of adult women affected with pelvic organ prolapse, have significant impact on their quality of life and emotional well-being. Epidemiologic survey of the United States showed that pelvic organs prolapse (POP) becomes more prevalent as the population age advances [1]. Women have 11.1% lifetime risk of undergoing surgery for prolapse by age 80 [2] and a 30% risk of reoperation over a period of 4 years [3].

Pelvic organ prolapse is defined as the descent of the anterior, posterior, and/or apical vaginal compartment(s) with protrusion of one or more pelvic organs (e.g. bladder, uterus,

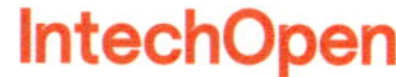

post-hysterectomy vaginal cuff, small bowel, or rectum) into the vagina [4]. These pathological changes are due to loss of structural support to pelvic organs resulting in an impact on women's quality of life. They arise because of injury and deterioration of the muscles, nerves, and connective tissue that support the pelvic floor and its contents.

Despite the high prevalence of POP, current treatment options remain suboptimal and do not address the underlying mechanisms of disease. Therefore, without improving our understanding of the pathophysiology of POP, treatment options and prevention of recurrence of POP would be limited. It is important to understand the pelvic floor support and the risk factors leading to POP. This chapter would include a review of pelvic floor support and the pathophysiology of POP.

2. Functional anatomy

Pelvic floor support includes:

1. Bony pelvis.
2. Subperitoneal connective tissue retinaculum and the broad ligament, including smooth muscle component and round ligament.
3. Cardinal and uterosacral ligaments complex.
4. Para vaginal attachments of the vaginal sulci to the arcus tendineus.
5. Urogenital diaphragm, including the pubourethrovaginal ligaments.
6. Pelvic diaphragm.
7. Fascia of denonvilliers.
8. Perineal body.

2.1. Bony pelvis

The support mechanism of Pelvic floor is provided by the complex and dynamic interactions of the muscles and connective tissues attachments within the bony pelvis. The bony pelvis provides fixed attachment to pelvic soft tissues and it consists of the two hip bones which made up of illium, ischium and pubis, anteriorly fused with each other at pubic symphysis and the sacrum posteriorly. The pelvis has divided into the false (or greater) pelvis and the true (or lesser) pelvis by the iliopectineal line, coursing along the superior edge of the superior pubic ramus, and circumferentially forms the pelvic brim. Within the true pelvis are the sacrotuberous and sacrospinous ligaments, contribute significant stability of the pelvis. The lesser pelvis is the narrower continuation of the greater pelvis inferiorly and its inferior pelvic outlet is closed by the pelvic floor.

2.2. Muscular support

2.2.1. Levator ani

Levator ani muscles form the pelvic diaphragm, which provide the firm tissue support of the pelvic floor. These muscles are attached to the inner surface of the true pelvis form the muscular floor of the pelvis. Three components of the levator ani muscles recognized are pubococcygeus, iliococcygeus and puborectalis [5]. The **pubococcygeus**, also known as puboviseralis muscle, arises from the anterior portion of the arcus tendineus and the back of the body of the pubis and is inserted with other parts of levator ani as anococcygeal raphe which forms a hiatus or levator plate. Pubovisceralis is further divided into pubovaginalis, puboanalis, and puboperinealis muscles [6]. The fibers attached to the perineal body are puboperinealis and draw this structure toward the pubic symphysis. The fibers attached to the anus at the intersphincteric groove between the internal and external anal sphincter are puboanalis. It elevates the anus and along with the rest of the pubococcygeus and puborectalis fibers keep the urogenital hiatus closed. Pubovaginalis refers to the medial fibers of pubococcygeus that attach to the lateral walls of the vagina.

The iliococcygeus arises from the arcus tendineus of the levator ani to the ischial spine and inserted into anococcygeal raphe. The puborectalis fibers of the levator ani (LA) muscle arises on lowest portion of pubic symphysis. It passes downward and backward on either side of vagina and fuses behind the rectum and form U-shaped muscular sling encircling the junction between the rectum and anus.

2.2.2. Coccygeus muscle

It forms the most posterior division of levator ani, arises from ischial spine and inserted into coccyx and lower sacrum. The piriformis and obturator internus form the posterolateral pelvic walls. The piriformis arises from the anterior and lateral surface of the sacrum and leaves the pelvis through the greater sciatic foramen, inserted to the greater trochanter of the femur. The obturator internus muscle arises from the ilium and ischium pelvic surfaces. It leaves the pelvis through the lesser sciatic foramen and inserted to the greater trochanter of the femur. The piriformis and obturator internus function as an external hip rotator.

2.3. Facial support

Endopelvic is composed of loose arrangements of collagen, elastin, and adipose tissue and condenses to form cardinal and uterosacral ligaments.

2.3.1. The ATLA

Arcus tendineous levator ani, dense connective tissue structure courses along the medial surface of the obturator internus muscle, serves as the point of origin for parts of the levator ani muscles (iliococcygeus). ATLA extends anteriorly from pubic tubercle to ischial spines posteriorly. The arcus tendineous fascia pelvis (ATFP), a thickening of fascia covering the medial aspect of the iliococcygeus muscles, extends from the inner surface of the superior pubic rami to the ischial spines. It provides lateral attachment point for the proximal rectovaginal septum and pubocervical fascia [7].

2.3.2. *Urogenital diaphragm*

The urogenital diaphragm, a dense fibromuscular sheet is like sandwich and composed of superior and inferior fascial layers separated from one another by (compressor urethra and urethrovaginal sphincter muscles), the deep transverse perineal muscles. It attaches laterally to the ishiopubic rami and medially to the distal third of the vagina and to the perineal body. In standing position, urogenital diaphragm is almost horizontal and its fixation to perineal body contributes to the support of urethra and vesicourethral junction [5].

2.3.3. *Perineal body*

The perineal body is a pyramidal fibromuscular elastic structure found between the distal third of the posterior vaginal wall and the anus on a line between the ischial tuberosity. The perineal body apex is continuous with the rectovaginal septum (the fascia of Denonvilliers) and it extends 2–3 cm above the hymeneal ring.

2.3.4. *Cardinal and uterosacral ligaments complex*

The parametria attaches lateral to the uterus is known as the cardinal and uterosacral ligament complex. They form three dimensional complex attaching the lower uterine segment, cervix and upper vagina with sacrum and pelvic side walls. This complex maintains vaginal length and keeps the vaginal axis horizontal. The uterosacral ligament also provides suspension and assist in maintaining the position of the uterus and upper vagina over the levator plate.

Using 3D stress magnetic resonance imaging (MRI) in vivo, dynamic of the cardinal and uterosacral ligament for apical support with and without Valsalva have been explored. [8]. These imaging techniques continue to enhance our knowledge of the strain and lengthening of these structures, which in turn, may help in determining the nature and direction of apical support loss.

3. Subdivision of pelvic floor

Anterior compartment is bordered by pubic symphysis ventrally, levator Ani laterally and perineal membrane caudally.

Posterior compartment has sacrum and coccyx dorsally, levator ani muscles laterally and caudally. Rectovaginal fascia constitutes an incomplete layer ventrocranially. Ventrocaudal border is composed by the perineal body.

Middle compartment has no distinct borders described ventrally. Laterally there are components of levator ani muscles and the perineal body caudally. Rectovaginal fascia constitutes the dorsal border [9].

http://dx.doi.org/10.5772/intechopen.76629

4. Pathogenesis

4.1. Risk factors of POP

4.1.1. Age

Age has been recognized as an intrinsic factor in the development of pelvic floor dysfunction and most consensuses in favor that it has a role in the etiology of female pelvic organ prolapse (POP) [10]. With advancing age, incidence and prevalence of POP increases. The relative prevalence of POP increased by about 40% with every decade of life, as demonstrated by a cross-sectional study of 1004 women (age 18–83 years) who attended their yearly examination [11].

Age and POP relation is hypothesized to be secondary to numerous factors including physiologic changes of the pelvic floor components and decline in estrogen during the postmenopausal period with advance age. This hypothesis is supported by Swift et al. study showing an increase in the odds ratio for pelvic prolapse from 1.04 to 1.46 for a change in 10 years of age [11].

4.1.2. Pregnancy and childbirth

There are hormonal induced physiological changes that occur in pelvic floor musculature and connective tissue during pregnancy. These alterations are vital for preparing the body to adjust the pelvic floor for vaginal birth. High level progesterone affects the pelvic floor by causing smooth muscle-relaxation and antagonizes estrogen effects.

Changes in biomechanical properties of the vaginal wall have been studied in fibulin-5 knockout mice (Fbln5$^{-/-}$) with and without prolapse [12]. He demonstrated that pregnant vaginal wall has increased distensibility, and decreased stiffness as compare to nonpregnant. The causative links between childbirth and prolapse have shown by various epidemiological and observational cohort studies [13, 14]. The pelvic structures affected by traumatic events are levator ani muscle complex, the pelvic nerves, the pelvic fascial structures and the anal sphincter.

Pregestational body mass index (BMI), BMI at term, duration of the first and second stages of labor, operative delivery, perineal lacerations, weight of the newborn and epidural analgesia are reported pregnancy related risk factors [14]. There is increased prevalence of true rectocele after vaginal childbirth as proven by many studies. Rectocele may be due to damage of the rectovaginal septum and Denonvillier's fascia in the posterior compartment [15]. Obstructed defaecation and pelvic organ prolapse are strongly associated with posterior compartment defects [16].

4.1.3. Raised intra-abdominal pressure

Chronically raised intra-abdominal pressure such as chronic constipation, higher body mass index (BMI), chronic cough, and repetitive heavy weight lifting seems to play a role in POP pathogenesis.

Morbid obesity was associated with 40% increase in the occurrence of uterine prolapse, 75% with rectocele and 57% with cystocele [17]. Five year follow up data [18] showed an increase in the risk for both anatomical and functional recurrence after vaginal surgery for POP in women with high body weight (>65 kg). Kuldish et al. studied the relationship between risk of prolapse progression in overweight and obese women compared with women with a normal BMI and found an increased by 32 and 48% for cystocele, by 37 and 58% for rectocele and by 43 and 69% for uterine prolapse [19]. Therefore it has been suggested that weight loss might help to prevent further progression and worsening of symptoms of prolapse and in reducing the post-surgical morbidity associated with obesity and prolapse surgery.

4.1.4. Previous pelvic organ surgery

Risk of subsequent pelvic organ prolapse is increased by hysterectomy however it takes years for development of symptomatic prolapse [20]. The mean interval between hysterectomy and surgery for pelvic organ prolapse in those who developed the prolapse was 19.3 years [21]. This occurs due to disruption of endopelvic fascia, uterosacral-cardinal ligament support and local nerve supply.

4.2. Pelvic floor defects

DeLancey [22] has described vaginal connective tissue support of the pelvis into three levels (**Figure 1**) that help to understand various clinical manifestations of pelvic organ support dysfunction. Level I, II and III representing apical, midvaginal and distal support respectively. Level I support is provided by cardinal and uterosacral ligament complex that suspends the vagina by attaching it to the pelvic side wall and is the most cephalad supporting structures.

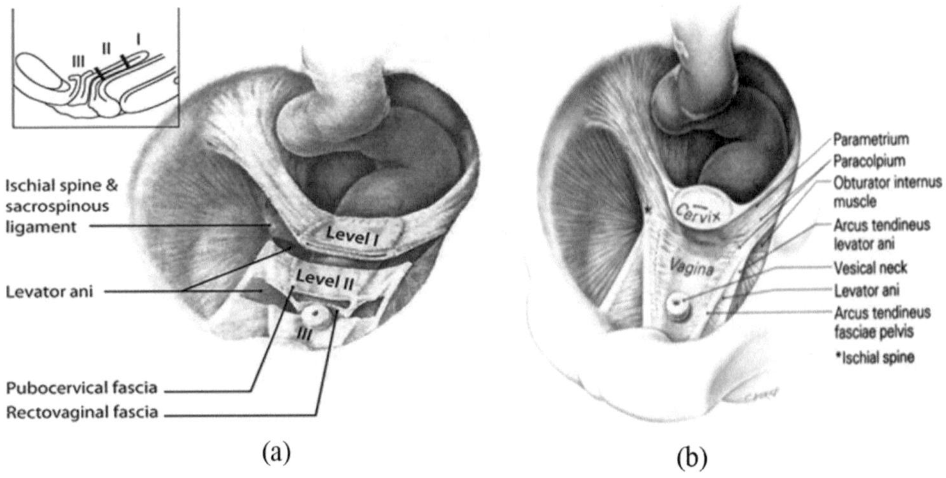

Figure 1. (A) In level I, paracolpium suspends vagina from the lateral pelvic walls. In level II, the vagina is attached to arcus tendineus of pelvic fascia and superior fascia of levator ani muscles. (B) Vagina and supportive structures drawn from dissection of a 56-year-old cadaver after hysterectomy: The bladder has been removed above the vesical neck. Paracolpium extends along the lateral wall of vagina. Reprinted, with permission, from DeLancey [22].

http://dx.doi.org/10.5772/intechopen.76629

In the middle vaginal portion, the vagina attaches laterally to the arcus tendineus and fascia of the levator ani muscles which stretches it transversely between the bladder and the rectum. The bladder support is provided by pubocervical fascia and its attachment through the endopelvic fascia to the pelvic side wall. Similarly, rectovaginal fascia forms the support of rectum and prevents it from protruding forward. The lower third of vagina fuses with the perineal membrane, levator ani muscles and perineal body and provided level III support.

4.2.1. *Compartments defects*

4.2.2. *Middle compartment defect*

According to the Integral Theory [23],the support to the upper vagina is provided by pericervical ring, form by pubocervical fascia (anteriorly), cardinal ligaments (laterally), uterosacral ligaments (posterolateral), and the rectovaginal fascia (posteriorly). The pelvic organs are suspended by three suspensory ligaments pubourethral (PUL), cardinal/uterosacral, and arcus tendineus fascia pelvis from the pelvic brim. Three directional muscle forces tension the organs to give them position, shape, and strength. The pelvic organs are opened or closed by neurologically coordinated forward and backward muscle forces contracting against these ligaments. Laxity or damage of these ligaments may nullify the muscle forces causing POP, urinary and bowel dysfunctions. Apical or middle compartment prolapse occurs, when support at bladder base is lost contributing to stress and urgency urinary symptoms, as support is provided by cervical ring [24].

On physical examination, detachment of this support may be recognized by assessing mobility and descent of the cervix and bulging of the anterior or posterior fornices. According to International Federation of Gynecology and Obstetrics (FIGO) [25] working group the reasons for apical descent are (1) the loss of apical support for the cardinal/uterosacral ligament complex, and (2) birth-related levator ani muscle injury.

Pelvic organ prolapse is believed to be associated with some degree of cervical elongation, possibly due to the increasing pressures causing downward displacement and hypertrophy of the cervix. Cervical lengths in women with and without Prolapse has been compared by Berger and Associates using pelvic MRI [26], and found that the amount of cervical elongation appeared to increase with greater degrees of uterine descent. Women with prolapse have 36.4% longer cervices than women without prolapse. However, it is difficult to assess clinically the cervical elongation and its significance is undetermined. The pelvic organ prolapse quantification (POP-Q) [27] examination allows in relation to fixed anatomic landmarks to evaluate the stages of prolapse in distinct compartments. Hypertrophic cervical elongation was defined as the difference between point C and point D of POP-Q as greater than 8 cm [28].

4.2.3. *Anterior compartment defect*

In maintaining bladder position, anterior vaginal wall support has a major role. The main structures involved are the anterior vaginal wall, pubocervical fascia, arcus tendineus fasciae pelvis (ATFP), arcus tendineus levator ani (ATLA), endopelvic fascia, and levator ani muscle.

The anterior compartment receives level I support at the pericervical ring whereas level II support is provided at the mid portion of anterior vagina which is attached laterally to the arcus tendineus fascia of the pelvic sidewall. The ATFPs act as suspension cables on either side of the vagina and bladder, harbor them to the pelvic wall and its detachment induces pelvic imbalance that may lead to lateral cystocele.

Petros described that bladder is supported anteriorly by the pubovesical ligaments and posteriorly by the cervical ring and laterally by the endopelvic fascia and ATFP [29]. The Pubocervical fascia is the main ventral support structure of the bladder, according to Petros. And disruption in pubocervical fascia results in cystocele. Level III (fusion) support at the distal third of the anterior compartment constitutes by fusion of the pubocervical fascia to the perineal membrane, perineal body, and levator ani muscles [30]. Although, controversy over the existence of a separate layer of fascia between the bladder and vagina. However, histologic studies of the anterior vaginal wall have failed to validate a separate layer of fascia between the vagina and the bladder [31]. Numerous cadaveric studies have demonstrated that the vesicovaginal space consists of fibroadipose tissue containing nerves and vascular channels [32] hence it has been recommended to used term "vaginal muscularis" or "fibromuscular wall instead of using the term pubocervical or pubovesical fascia when describing the anterior vaginal wall tissue and support [33].

For the understanding of anterior compartment prolapse, different theories evolved with time. Richardson described areas of "breaks" in the "fascia" of the anterior vaginal wall, in the form of lateral paravaginal defects, transverse defect due to separation of the pubocervical fascia from the pericervical ring and, anteroposterior separation of fascia between bladder and vagina result in midline defect [34].

Petros' and DeLancey's anatomic/functional theories of bladder support structures discriminated three types of cystocele include apical, medial, and lateral or paravaginal [22, 29]. Apical cystocele is due to anatomic defect in the upper third of the vagina which include endopelvic fascia and DeLancey's level 1 ligament complex. Medial cystocele relates to the cervical ring defect. DeLancey found association between cervical-ring defect and high-grade cystocele by assessing anatomical lesions on MRI. Defects in Uterosacral ligaments and the Pubocervical fascia result in 75% of high-grade cystoceles. Lateral cystocele relate to both ligamentous and pelviperineal muscular defect which involves pubocervical fascia, the ATLA and the ATFP. Detachment of any of these bladder support result into lateral cystocele. Other factors such as obstructed voiding symptoms may be indicators of prolapse severity or absence of vaginal rugae also may suggest the location of certain anterior wall support defects [35].

Using biomechanical model, Chen and associates [36] analyzed the magnitude of anterior vaginal wall prolapse. They postulated that anterior vaginal prolapse dependent on the degree of impairment sustained by the pubovisceral muscle and the cardinal/uterosacral ligament complex under raised intra-abdominal pressure. They demonstrated the loss of support of the levator ani muscles leads to downward rotation of the levator plate (trap door opens), and widening of the urogenital hiatus., and worsening anterior vaginal wall prolapse, trap door theory effect.

4.2.4. Posterior compartment

Level III support of posterior vaginal wall is via fusion of the "rectovaginal fascia" to the perineal membrane, perineal body, and levator ani muscles and prevents rectum downward descent in this region. The middle third of the vaginal (Level II) support is through lateral endopelvic fascial attachments. Level I support shared with that of the anterior compartment (cardinal and uterosacral ligaments), where anterior and posterior vaginal walls abut.

The concepts on the mechanical support in the posterior compartment have been introduced by DeLancey [37]. According to that the pelvic floor closure by the puborectalis muscle contraction draws the posterior vaginal wall against the anterior vaginal wall, allowing for balanced pressures on either wall upon Valsalva. With the levator ani muscles injury, that created an unbalanced downward force on the posterior compartment, result in tension on the structures associated with level II support.

The posterior paravaginal defects due to loss of lateral attachments to the rectovaginal fascia whereas detachments of the distal "rectovaginal fascia" to the perineal body, which may evident as a perineal bulge or "low" posterior wall prolapse. In contrast high posterior wall defects are associated to loss of level I support to the pericervical ring and cardinal uterosacral complex.

4.2.5. Alteration of collagen and smooth muscles of the vagina

Comprehensively, it has been reviewed that abnormal synthesis or degradation of collagen and elastin fibers of the vaginal wall contributes to the pathophysiology of prolapse [38].

The pelvic organs are invested by connective tissues that provide the anatomic support of the pelvis and its contents. Histologically the normal vaginal wall comprises of four layers: a superficial non-keratinised stratified squamous epithelium; a subepithelial dense connective tissue layer composed primarily of collagen and elastin; muscularis; a layer of smooth muscle and adventitia, composed of loose connective tissue. The subepithelium and muscularis together give the tensile strength to the vaginal wall. The connective tissues of the vagina and supportive tissues comprise predominantly of fibrillar component (collagen and elastin) embedded in a non-fibrillar component (noncollagenous glycoproteins, hyaluronan, and proteoglycans), with the exception of the arcus tendineous, contain a significant amount of smooth muscle [39].

Collagen types I, III are the main structural constituents of vaginal epithelium and endopelvic fascia. Type I collagen confers strength to tissues associated with ligamentous tissue while type III contributes to elasticity found in loose areolar tissue, which makes up the vaginal wall adventitia and surrounds the pelvic organs. The ratio of collagen I to III is an indicator of tensile strength: the higher the amount of collagen type I, the higher is the mechanical strength. Balance is precisely maintained between quality and quantity of collagen through synthesis, posttranslational modification, and degradation and its deficiencies has been associated with the development of pelvic organ prolapses.

The matrix metalloproteinases (MMPs) is proteolytic enzyme involved in both physiological and pathological tissue remodeling in women with and without prolapse. Women predispose to prolapse with an excessive tendency toward connective tissue degradation. The proteolytic activity in turn is regulated by inhibitors, TIMPs who bind with MMPS and inhibit its activity. In comparing women without prolapse, prolapse showed higher expression of MMP-2 mRNA with a concurrent decrease in the inhibitor TIMP-2 [40].

On comparing pre and postmenopausal women with and without prolapse, Takano [41] found decreased in amount of collagen with prolapse irrespective of menopausal status. Moalli et al. [42] demonstrated an increased in collagen III in vaginal subepithelium and muscularis in women with prolapse independent of age and parity. There is also Increase in collagen III content in the uterosacral and cardinal ligaments in women with prolapse [43]. The Moalli's group [44] analyzed a reduced in the ratio of collagen I/(III + V) is associated with menopause and with used of hormonal therapy restoration of this ratio to menarche level. This suggested the biomechanical properties of the supportive tissues of the vagina may improve with used of sex steroid hormones. Thus the increased stretchability and distensibility and decline in tensile strength associated with a higher content of collagen III are likely to contribute to the progression of POP.

5. Conclusion

Better understanding of pelvic functional anatomy, helps in understanding the pathophysiology of POP. The major support is by the levator ani muscles, pelvic connective tissue, vaginal walls and defects in these structures results in the genesis of pelvic floor dysfunction. Although the etiology of POP is multifactorial, but vaginal delivery is recognized as the strongest risk factor by many epidemiologic studies. However more research in these areas will, in turn lead to development of preventative strategies and better treatment modalities in women at high risk for the development of POP.

Author details

Lubna Razzak

Address all correspondence to: lubna.razzak@aku.edu

Aga Khan University, Karachi, Pakistan

References

[1] National Center for Health Statistics (US). Health, United States: With Special Feature on Medical Technology; 2009

[2] Olsen AL, Smith VJ, Bergstrom JO, Colling JC, Clark AL. Epidemiology of surgically managed pelvic organ prolapse and urinary incontinence. Obstetrics & Gynecology. Apr 1, 1997;**89**(4):501-506

[3] Boyles SH, Weber AM, Meyn L. Procedures for pelvic organ prolapse in the United States, 1979-1997. American Journal of Obstetrics and Gynecology. Jan 31, 2003;**188**(1):108-115

[4] DeLancey JO. The hidden epidemic of pelvic floor dysfunction: Achievable goals for improved prevention and treatment. American Journal of Obstetrics and Gynecology. May 31, 2005;**192**(5):1488-1495

[5] Corton MM. Aspects of gynecologic surgery. Chapter 38. Anatomy. In: Hoffman BL, Schorge JO, Schaffer JI, et al, editors. Williams Gynecology. 2nd ed. New York: McGraw-Hill Medical; 2012. pp. 917-947

[6] Kearney R, Sawhney R, DeLancey JO. Levator ani muscle anatomy evaluated by origin-insertion pairs. Obstetrics and Gynecology. Jul 2004;**104**(1):168

[7] Albright TS, Gehrich AP, Davis GD, et al. Arcus tendineus fascia pelvis: A further understanding. American Journal of Obstetrics and Gynecology. Sep 30, 2005;**193**(3):677-681

[8] Luo J, Betschart C, Chen L, et al. Using stress MRI to analyze the 3D changes in apical ligament geometry from rest to maximal Valsalva: A pilot study. International Urogynecology Journal. Feb 1, 2014;**25**(2):197-203

[9] Santoro GA, Sultan AH. Pelvic floor anatomy and imaging. In: Seminars in Colon and Rectal Surgery. Vol. 27, No. 1. Elsevier; Mar 1, 2016. pp. 5-14

[10] Jelovsek JE, Maher C, Barber MD. Pelvic organ prolapse. The Lancet. Mar 30, 2007; **369**(9566):1027-1038

[11] Swift S et al. Pelvic organ support study (POSST): The distribution, clinical definition, and epidemiologic condition of pelvic organ support defects. American Journal of Obstetrics and Gynecology. Mar 31, 2005;**192**(3):795-806

[12] Rahn DD et al. Biomechanical properties of the vaginal wall: Effect of pregnancy, elastic fiber deficiency, and pelvic organ prolapse. American Journal of Obstetrics and Gynecology. May 31, 2008;**198**(5):590-e1

[13] O'Boyle AL et al. Pelvic organ support in nulliparous pregnant and nonpregnant women: A case control study. American Journal of Obstetrics and Gynecology. Jul 31, 2002;**187**(1):99-102

[14] Bertozzi S et al. Impact of episiotomy on pelvic floor disorders and their influence on women's wellness after the sixth month postpartum: A retrospective study. BMC Women's Health. Apr 18, 2011;**11**(1):12

[15] Dietz H, Steensma AB. The role of childbirth in the aetiology of rectocele. BJOG: An International Journal of Obstetrics & Gynaecology. Mar 1, 2006;**113**(3):264-267

[16] Dietz HP, Korda A. Which bowel symptoms are most strongly associated with as rectocele? Australian and New Zealand Journal of Obstetrics and Gynaecology. Dec 1, 2005;**45**(6):505-508

[17] Hendrix SL, Clark A, Nygaard I, et al. Pelvic organ prolapse in the Women's Health Initiative: Gravity and gravidity. American Journal of Obstetrics and Gynecology. Jun 30, 2002;**186**(6):1160-1166

[18] Diez-Itza I, Aizpitarte I, Becerro A. Risk factors for the recurrence of pelvic organ prolapse after vaginal surgery: A review at 5 years after surgery. International Urogynecology Journal. Nov 1, 2007;**18**(11):1317

[19] Kudish BI et al. Effect of weight change on natural history of pelvic organ prolapse. Obstetrics and Gynecology.. Jan 2009;**113**(1):81

[20] Moalli PA, Ivy SJ, Meyn LA, Zyczynski HM. Risk factors associated with pelvic floor disorders in women undergoing surgical repair. Obstetrics & Gynecology. May 31, 2003;**101**(5):869-874

[21] Clark AL, Gregory T, Smith VJ, Edwards R. Epidemiologic evaluation of reoperation for surgically treated pelvic organ prolapse and urinary incontinence. American Journal of Obstetrics and Gynecology. Nov 30, 2003;**189**(5):1261-1267

[22] DeLancey JO. Anatomie aspects of vaginal eversion after hysterectomy. American Journal of Obstetrics and Gynecology. Jun 1, 1992;**166**(6):1717-1728

[23] Liedl B et al. Update of the integral theory and system for management of pelvic floor dysfunction in females. European Urology Supplements. Apr 1, 2018;**17**(3):100-8

[24] Petros PE, Ulmsten UI. An integral theory of female urinary incontinence. Acta Obstetricia et Gynecologica Scandinavica. Jan 1, 1990;**69**(S153):7-31

[25] Betschart C et al. Management of apical compartment prolapse (uterine and vault prolapse): A FIGO Working Group report. Neurourology and Urodynamics. Feb 1, 2017;**36**(2):507-513

[26] Berger MB, Ramanah R, Guire KE, et al. Is cervical elongation associated with pelvic organ prolapse? International Urogynecology Journal. Aug 1, 2012;**23**(8):1095-1103

[27] Bump RC, Mattiasson A, Bo K, et al. The standardization of terminology of female pelvic organ prolapse and pelvic floor dysfunction. American Journal of Obstetrics and Gynecology. Jul 31, 1996;**175**(1):10-17

[28] Ibeanu OA, Chesson RR, Sandquist D, et al. Hypertrophic cervical elongation: Clinical and histological correlations. International Urogynecology Journal. Aug 1, 2010; **21**(8):995-1000

[29] Papa Petros PE, Ulmsten UI. An integral theory of female urinary incontinence: Experimental and clinical considerations. Acta obstetricia et gynecologica Scandinavica. Supplement. 1990;**153**:7-31

[30] Ricci JV, Thom CH. The myth of a surgically useful fascia in vaginal plastic reconstructions. Quarterly Review of Surgery. Dec 1954;**11**(4):253

[31] Tamilselvi A. Current concepts in pelvic anatomy. In: Principles and Practice of Urogynaecology. India: Springer; 2015. pp. 3-15

[32] Weber AM, Walters MD. Anterior vaginal prolapse: review of anatomy and techniques of surgical repair. Obstetrics & Gynecology. Feb 1, 1997;**89**(2):311-318

[33] Corton MM. Anatomy of pelvic floor dysfunction. Obstetrics and Gynecology Clinics of North America. Sep 30, 2009;**36**(3):401-419

[34] Maldonado PA, Wai CY. Pelvic organ prolapse: New concepts in pelvic floor anatomy. Obstetrics and Gynecology Clinics. Mar 1, 2016;**43**(1):15-26

[35] Whiteside JL, Barber MD, Paraiso MF, Walters MD. Vaginal rugae: Measurement and significance. Climacteric. Mar 1, 2005;**8**(1):71-75

[36] Chen L, Ashton-Miller JA, Hsu Y, DeLancey JO. Interaction between apical supports and levator ani in anterior vaginal support: Theoretical analysis. Obstetrics and Gynecology. Aug 2006;**108**(2):324

[37] DeLancey JO. Structural anatomy of the posterior pelvic compartment as it relates to rectocele. American Journal of Obstetrics and Gynecology. Apr 30, 1999;**180**(4):815-823

[38] Kerkhof MH, Hendriks L, Brölmann HA. Changes in connective tissue in patients with pelvic organ prolapse—A review of the current literature. International Urogynecology Journal. Apr 1, 2009;**20**(4):461

[39] Alperin M, Moalli PA. Remodeling of vaginal connective tissue in patients with prolapse. Current Opinion in Obstetrics and Gynecology. Oct 1, 2006;**18**(5):544-550

[40] Liang CC et al. Expression of matrix metalloproteinase-2 and tissue inhibitors of metalloproteinase-1 (TIMP-1, TIMP-2 and TIMP-3) in women with uterine prolapse but without urinary incontinence. European Journal of Obstetrics & Gynecology and Reproductive Biology. Nov 30, 2010;**153**(1):94-98

[41] Takano CC et al. Analysis of collagen in parametrium and vaginal apex of women with and without uterine prolapse. International Urogynecology Journal. Nov 1, 2002;**13**(6): 342-345

[42] Moalli PA et al. Remodeling of vaginal connective tissue in patients with prolapse. Obstetrics & Gynecology. Nov 1, 2005;**106**(5, Part 1):953-963

[43] Gabriel B et al. Uterosacral ligament in postmenopausal women with or without pelvic organ prolapse. International Urogynecology Journal. Dec 1, 2005;**16**(6):475-479

[44] Moalli PA et al. Regulation of matrix metalloproteinase expression by estrogen in fibroblasts that are derived from the pelvic floor. American Journal of Obstetrics and Gynecology. Jul 31, 2002;**187**(1):72-79

Chapter 3

Effects of Posture and Gravity on Pelvic Organ Prolapse

Marwa Abdulaziz, Lynn Stothers and
Andrew Macnab

Additional information is available at the end of the chapter

http://dx.doi.org/10.5772/intechopen.77040

Abstract

Female pelvic floor dysfunction occurs when the integrity of the pelvic floor muscles is compromised and impacts the position and function of the pelvic organs. Physicians use international guidelines to evaluate and treat women for POP taking into account that posture and gravity impact pelvic organ position, and degree of prolapse. Our clinical focuses on the description of surface anatomy. This examination alone is insufficient. Although imaging is recommended, the modalities currently available are recognized to have flaws. MRI is performed in the supine position regardless the effect of posture and gravity on POP. A literature search was performed using databases, searching MEDLINE and PubMed using the key terms ultrasound, MRI, and CT. We describe use of a new protocol and advanced technique to evaluate the changes of POP in different positions using open MRI (MRO). POP patients underwent MRO imaging of the pelvic floor using a 0.5 T MRO scanner. The extent of displacement of prolapsed organs was determined using validated reference lines drawn on the mid-sagittal images. Manual segmentation and surface modeling were used to construct the 3D models. MRO offers new levels of anatomic detail; 3D sequences based on 2D images are an additional refinement.

Keywords: magnetic resonance imaging, upright open MRI, ultrasound, CT scan, 3D computer generated image

1. Introduction

Female pelvic floor dysfunction is a widespread condition where the associated symptoms of urinary and fecal incontinence negatively impact the quality of life of many women. The life time risk of surgery for pelvic organ prolapse (POP) in women is estimated as 10–20%.

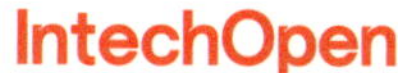

Despite the pervasiveness, our information about the etiology and pathophysiology of female pelvic floor dysfunction is limited, as evaluation is primarily based on physical examination using international guidelines [1]. Imaging is recommended in addition, but current methods are not able to assess the effects of posture and gravity, factors recognized to impact pelvic organ position, pelvic floor muscle integrity, degree of prolapse, and symptom severity. Importantly, the degree of prolapse may be worse after a lengthy time in the upright position and better when gravity is not a factor, e.g., when lying in the supine position.

The first imaging of pelvic floor dysfunction was done in the 1920s [2]. Radiological techniques were first used to show bladder manifestations and subsequently for central and posterior compartment prolapse [3]. The advent of B-mode real-time ultrasound presented a technique that allowed for a clear image by the transperineal or the vaginal route [4, 5]. Later, magnetic resonance imaging (MRI) emerged as an option. Although MRI provided imaging of ligamentous and muscular pelvic floor structures in fine detail, the cost of imaging, access problems, and restriction to imaging patients in the supine position have obstructed its general acceptance [6].

Most recently, upright open MRI has become available, which allows the patient to be imaged when sitting or standing as well as supine [7]. We have conducted research literature search that has allowed a protocol to be developed for using upright open MRI to more comprehensively evaluate patients with POP and demonstrate where posture and gravity have impact on organ positions and symptom severity.

2. Pelvic organ prolapse

Pelvic organ prolapse (POP) is a prevalent condition affecting up to 50% of parous women; it most often presents with symptoms of urinary incontinence [8]. Traditionally, gynecologists identify prolapse by using a simple clinical staging system (stages 0 to III or IV), with 0 indicating normal conditions and III or IV denoting full organ prolapse or vaginal eversion fOP-Q staging for POP (POP-Q).

The accuracy of staging is important, as the treatment or surgery recommended to the patient is based on the staging of their POP. However, surgical repair of prolapse has a failure rate as high as 30%, and this is probably due to current pre-surgical evaluation providing incomplete assessment of the extent of the underlying structural changes causing the prolapse, resulting in incomplete repair. For instance, the levator ani muscle complex plays an important role in pelvic organ support. Evaluation of the integrity of this element of the pelvic structures is particularly difficult, and clinical examination alone is often insufficient [9].

Physicians assess patients using guidelines from organizations such as the International Urogynecological Association (IUGA) and International Continence Society (ICS) to evaluate women for POP and define treatment options to address the associated urinary and fecal incontinence.

The guidelines recommend steps for physical examination of symptomatic women which recognize that whether the patient is standing, sitting, or lying affects the position of the pelvic organs and the type, occurrence, and severity of symptoms. Hence, examination is done with the woman's bladder (and preferably rectum) empty, using the left lateral (Sims), or supine, standing, or lithotomy position, depending on which best demonstrates POP in that patient, and which the patient confirms is the maximal extent she has perceived. Forced expiration against a closed glottis (Valsalva) increases the accuracy of diagnosis CHANGE REFERENCE to a recent one/update the reference [10].

However, problematically, not all women can Valsalva effectively or tolerate examination when upright, and the guidelines acknowledge that "the more complicated the history and the more extensive and/or invasive the proposed therapy, the more complete the examination needs to be" [11]. Hence, further evaluation using imaging modalities is recommended when the appropriate indication(s) are present, with imaging highly recommended in specific situations. (IUGA) Imaging modalities employed currently include 2D and 3D ultrasound (US), computed tomography (CT), and magnetic resonance imaging (MRI).

Current research on the association between childbirth-related pelvic floor muscle trauma and female POP provides an example of how imaging can aid better understanding of the pathophysiology of pelvic floor dysfunction [12–15], allowing primary (inflatable balloon device) [16] and secondary (surgical repair) prevention trials, and if all goes well resulting in efficient treatment based on translational research [17, 18].

Clinical examination focuses primarily on surface anatomy, which alone is not able to fully detect the extent of the underlying structural abnormalities. For example, prolapse of the posterior vagina, which is most prevalent in women with symptoms of prolapse and obstructed defecation is called "rectocele", and it occurs in at least five distinct anatomical forms that are hard to define without imaging [19]. Improved imaging of the pelvic floor to quantify and determine pelvic floor support has been identified as an important method to improve our understanding of POP, aid our ability to perform surgical repair, and to define the causes for surgical failure [20]. However, the position of the levator ani within the pelvic cavity, encircled as this structure is by the bony pelvis, and its shape, make direct imaging complex.

The differences between cystocele, enterocele, and rectocele are also difficult to determine with physical examination and are much better evaluated with imaging. Imaging also can discover unsuspected defects like enteroceles and sigmoidoceles [21]. The discovery rate of enteroceles is less with physical examination than with imaging; this is because of the misdiagnosis of enteroceles as rectoceles [22].

The role of imaging is to identify clinically suspected problems, discriminate between different anatomic defects, and define unsuspected problems in pelvic floor support. In patients with non-specific clinical findings, MRI can provide additional information to assess the need for surgical repair of the pelvic floor [21].

3. Patient positioning

The relevance of posture on the extent of POP and severity of associated symptoms is well recognized. However, investigation of the influence of the body posture on pelvic floor pathologies and defecation has been done in only a few studies. Dynamic pelvic floor imaging is performed in the supine position with patients lying in a closed-configuration MR scanner [23]. The principal reason for this is the limitation on imaging to the supine position. Lying supine is also comfortable for most patients, and this technique has been simple to standardize. However, in POP, posture and gravity impact pelvic organ position, pelvic floor muscle integrity, degree of prolapse, and symptom severity. Indeed, the degree of prolapse may be worse after a lengthy time in the upright position and better when gravity is not a factor, e.g., when lying in the supine position [10]. Hence, one could question if measurement in the lying position is valid for assessment of muscle function or the evaluation of patients who are symptomatic in the standing position [24].

Additionally, gravity and body weight contribute to pelvic organ muscle contractile features when standing [25]. It is likely that complex factors related to upright posture that produce more contractility over pre-loaded and/or pre-activated muscles come into play, as the weight of pelvic organs and gravity are contributing forces affecting the pelvic floor. This may explain why digital muscle testing and squeeze-pressure readings can be lower in the standing position. However, it is not known exactly which components of pelvic organ muscle activation — squeeze or lift — are influenced by alterations in posture.

Hypothetically speaking, the dynamics of the whole pelvic floor may be modified (or the squeeze and the elevation components might be influenced variously) owing to different effects such as descent of the pelvic organs when standing, different tensions on fascia and ligaments, alteration in resting length and tone of the contractile elements, and other factors.

It is well known that being upright results in a displacement of the pelvic organs and the pelvic organs muscle as compared with being supine [24, 26]. The full bladder is less mobile than the empty organ this factor may prohibit complete pelvic organ prolapse. In the standing orientation, the bladder is situated lower at rest but descends about as far in a lying patient on a Valsalva maneuver [27]. Dietz and Clarke [27] in their population of 132 patients with pelvic floor dysfunction found a 5-mm difference in the resting level of the bladder neck between supine and standing as measured by transperineal ultrasound. The only study comparing MRI in sitting and lying positions found that they were equally efficient in recognizing clinically relevant problems of the pelvic floor [28].

The position and eventual prolapse of pelvic organs is best visualized on MRI in the midsagittal plane. The imaging technique for the pelvic floor involves imaging several pelvic floor positions. Firstly, the position of the pelvic organs is assessed at rest. Then, the pelvic floor muscles images are recorded during squeezing to view the contractility and the strength of contraction of the pelvic floor. In the third phase, pelvic floor pathologies are assessed during straining and evacuation. In a recent study to view the full extent of pelvic floor pathologies, imaging was done during evacuation of a contrast agent; a number of pathologic conditions would have been missed if these defecation phase images had not been acquired [29].

4. Current imaging techniques

Evaluation using imaging modalities is recommended in international guidelines when the appropriate indication(s) are present, and imaging is highly recommended in specific situations [10]. Imaging modalities employed currently include 2D and 3D ultrasound, computed tomography, and magnetic resonance imaging.

4.1. Ultrasound

Imaging the pelvic floor in cases of dysfunction dates back to the 1920s [2]. Radiological techniques were used first to show changes in the bladder's location within the pelvis and subsequently to demonstrate central and posterior compartment prolapse. During the 1980s the advent of B-mode real-time ultrasound allowed a clear image to be obtained by the transperineal or the vaginal route [19].

Translabial ultrasound can define uterovaginal prolapse [30]. The inferior border of the symphysis pubis works as a line of reference against which the higher descent of bladder, uterus, culde sac, and rectal ampulla on Valsalva maneuver can be measured [30]. Ultrasound imaging for prolapse quantification is especially helpful in outcome evaluation after pelvic reconstructive surgery, both clinically and in a research context, and it has also led to a re-appraisal of what is meant by prolapse.

The structures used for evaluation of the three compartments are (a) the bladder neck or the leading edge of a cystocele for the anterior vaginal wall, (b) the cervix (or, within certain limitations, the pouch of Douglas) for the central compartment, and (c) the rectal ampulla for the posterior compartment. All these structures are imaged in real time in the mid-sagittal plane. An exception is a high undescended uterus that may be hidden by a rectocele [10]. Because of its non-invasive nature, ready availability, and lack of distortion, perineal or translabial ultrasound is now commonly applied in clinical practice [30], and almost all gynecologists and urologists are trained in its use [19].

Current developments such as the evaluation of levator ani muscle activity and prolapse and the use of color Doppler to define urine leakage are further promoting the clinical utility of ultrasound. Hopefully, improved standardization of parameters will facilitate the ability of clinicians and researchers to compare data [30].

Regardless of which technique is used to define descent of the pelvic organs, it is obvious that there is a large difference in pelvic organ mobility even in young nulliparous women. This difference may be partially genetic in origin. Ultrasound imaging permits quantification of the wide variation in pelvic organ mobility, which will make it easier to use molecular and population genetic approaches to assess the etiology of pelvic floor and bladder dysfunction [30].

It seems to be irrelevant with chapter title Ultrasound imaging of the pelvic floor is safer, lower in cost, and better at providing visualization of the pelvic floor structures in real time than MRI. This includes evaluation of levator function and dynamic changes during contraction and Valsalva [20]. As yet, there are no comparisons of pre- and postnatal results gained with MRI, possibly because of cost and logistic problems. However, such a comparison is available for many hundreds of women studied by 4D translabial ultrasound [2].

Disadvantages of ultrasound include that a large bowel-filled prolapse, i.e., an enterocele or rectocele, may cause incomplete imaging of the cervix and vault if these structures remain high. In addition, variable transducer pressure can result in an underestimation of severe prolapse. Procidentia or complete vaginal eversion prevents translabial imaging, and sometimes what appears to be anterior vaginal wall prolapse will turn out to be due to a urethral diverticulum [31, 32].

4.2. CT scan

CT is not usually recommended for imaging the pelvic floor because of the level of radiation required. However, this modality can offer accurate visualization of the pelvic soft tissue and bony structures and has been used to increase the diagnostic accuracy of pelvic floor anatomical disorders [1]. Although the soft tissue contrast with CT is inferior to that of MRI, the bladder, uterus, small bowel, peritoneal fat, and rectum are readily identified, and changes in position with the patient straining can be visualized. Additionally, the contour of the levator ani muscles can be evaluated effectively, and images of pelvic anatomy can be produced in multiple planes. Therefore, in patients who cannot tolerate MRI and in whom rapid noninvasive multiplanar assessment of the pelvis is desired, CT has a potential role. With recent scanners, tube output can be modified depending on the patient's body thickness, and this may help to decrease the radiation dose given. The pelvic floor and viscera can be visualized, and the addition of dynamic imaging can be applied to determine prolapse [33].

4.3. MRI

Techniques associated with urology have developed over the last 30 years. In the 1990s MR techniques were improved with rapid and strong gradients and higher readout bandwidth. The first study depicting the using of MR for imaging pelvic organ prolapse was by Yang et al.

The increasing availability of MRI has added the benefit of this form of diagnostic imaging to evaluation in urogynecology and female urology, with more studies being done every year [30]. With the option of cross-sectional imaging methods, MRI has emerged as an alternate method to fluoroscopy for assessing patients with pelvic organ prolapse [34].

Benefits of MRI include multiplanar imaging and superior soft tissue contrast, permitting evaluation of the pelvic floor levator ani muscle in detail. The anatomy of the levator ani is now known to be complex; it has been shown not to be a single muscle, being composed of two functional components that differ in thickness and function [20]. In addition, where there is organ prolapse, enhanced visualization of the rectovaginal space improves diagnosis of peritoneoceles and enteroceles and of the cervix clarifies cervical descent [33]. This allows demonstration of enterocele-type defects or peritoneoceles where there is just herniation of peritoneal fat and not bowel, comprehensive evaluation of the levator ani muscle, and visualization of the uterus.

The position and relationship of the pelvic organs are best visualized on MRI in the midsagittal plane. The imaging technique for the pelvic floor involves imaging in various pelvic floor positions. Firstly, the position of the pelvic organs is assessed at rest. Then, the pelvic floor muscles images are recorded during squeezing to view the contractility and the strength of contraction of the pelvic floor. In the third phase, pelvic floor pathologies are assessed during straining and evacuation. In a recent study to view the full extent of pelvic floor pathologies imaging was done during evacuation of a contrast agent; a number of pathologic conditions would have been missed if these defecation phase images had not been acquired [29].

Dynamic MRI techniques have been shown to be more sensitive than pelvic examination in evaluating and grading pelvic floor displacement in supine women and also for diagnosis of rectoceles [35, 42]. In the case of an anorectal problem, MR defecography can identify several components of pelvic floor dysfunction, including rectal descent, enterocele, anterior proctocele, and internal rectal prolapse [36].

The short acquisition time is relevant because patients do not need to keep on straining for more than 1 to 3 s. Patients are instructed in the Valsalva maneuver before the start of the examination, and instructions are repeated frequently during the imaging sequence [37, 38]. Dynamic sequences that permit the acquisition of images in 1 to 10 s are helpful to obtain maximal strain [39].

Sometimes, patients cannot tolerate MRI due to claustrophobia, general weakness, or the presence of medical equipment [33]. Positive elements of MRI include the fact that filling the bladder, the vagina, or the rectum does not seem to be a fundamental requirement because of to the high resolution of MRI, which prevents distorting the anatomy of the pelvic organs [40]. Also, in a research context, MRI is acceptable to asymptomatic volunteers [40].

The expense of MRI imaging and limited access to scanning facilities has impacted widespread application of this technology. Additionally, because of the dynamic nature of pelvic floor pathology, it is controversial whether even fast MRI imaging can capture reproducible results owing to the dissimilarity of Valsalva maneuvers between studies and possible variations in levator activity [10].

The physical features of MRI systems make it complicated for the operator to ensure efficient conduct of the required maneuvers by patients; over 50% of women do not achieve a proper pelvic floor contraction during examination, and a Valsalva is very often confounded by associated levator ani activation [41]. Without real-time imaging, these confounders cannot be controlled for [2] upright open MRI.

Importantly this provides the ability to replicate normal functional posture and enables the effects of gravity on prolapse to be evaluated for the first time [7]. In POP, posture and gravity impact pelvic organ position, pelvic floor muscle integrity, degree of prolapse, and symptom severity, and the degree of prolapse may be worse after time in the upright position and better when gravity is not a factor, e.g., when lying in the supine position [1]. Near-real-time sequences allow images to be obtained every 1.5 s. These can be stored and displayed on video, enabling a dynamic assessment of the pelvic floor from the resting position through straining and contraction [40]. The gynecologic literature proposes that straining in the lying position does not give sufficient deformity of the pelvic floor for accurate delineation of prolapse.

Upright open MRI allows visualization of all the pelvic organs and the pelvic floor support structures; obviously the technique combines the advance of allowing sitting and standing imaging with the known benefits of conventional MRI. We believe that the importance of this technique is that it enables comprehensive definition of the full extent of organ prolapse due to the effects of posture and gravity [40].

Upright open MRI is currently only available as a research entity. A new clinical protocol for MRO image capture of the female pelvis has been created and introduced into clinical practice. This provides enhanced anatomic definition and allows more comprehensive evaluation and staging.

5. Reference lines

Image interpretation from conventional and upright open MRI evaluates the three compartments of the pelvic floor [43]. The three compartments are evaluated for morphologic changes such as POP at various pelvic floor positions. To define the existence and descent of POP, the use of a point of reference is beneficial. Several points and lines of reference for measuring POP have been reported [44]. The more commonly used lines are the pubococcygeal line (PCL) and the mid-pubic line (MPL), both applied on midsagittal images. The PCL is the line drawn from the inferior part of the symphysis pubis to the last coccygeal joint. Extending the posterior portion of the PCL to the sacrococcygeal joint also has been proposed because there is movability of the coccyx with straining [21]. The MPL is a line extending along the long axis of the symphysis pubis. The PCL represents the levator plate, while the MPL correlates with the level of the hymen, which is the landmark applied for clinical staging [45]. To measure pelvic organ prolapse a perpendicular line is drawn from the reference line (PCL or MPL) to the bladder base (anterior compartment), the cervix or vaginal vault (middle compartment), and the anal rectal junction (ARJ) (posterior compartment) [23].

Another classification system, H line, M line, organ prolapse (HMO), has been proposed for measuring prolapse [35]. The H line is drawn from the pubis to the posterior anorectal junction and measures the levator hiatus width. Organ prolapse is measured relative to that line. The M line measures the descent of the levator plate from the pubococcygeal line. The angle of the levator plate relative to the pubococcygeal line and the width and part of the pelvic hiatus on axial images can be measured as well [22].

The choice of which reference line is used is mostly made by the radiologist and/or the referring clinician, as neither of the two lines has shown distinct superiority [44]. The PCL, however, is the most-used reference line, particularly by surgeons and gastroenterologists. The MPL is better known among urogynecologists, as it is compatible with their clinical staging system. Both reference lines display only moderate to poor agreement with clinical staging of pelvic organ prolapse [38]. This might be partly because anatomical landmarks used for MR measurements and for clinical examination differed in most of the studies [23]. Standards exist for diagnosing prolapse on physical examination [1]. Congruity between this clinical standard and MRI imaging analysis should be used to document the utility of MRI and the success of treatment [22].

However, different criteria are currently used for diagnosing prolapse on MRI. Most research that reported using the bony reference lines uses one of the following criteria: (a) descent of the bladder base more than 1 cm inferior to the pubococcygeal line, (b) position of the cervix or vaginal vault less than 1 cm over the PCL or below it, and (c) descent of the posterior compartment more than 2.5 cm below the PCL (International Urogynecological Association and International Continence Society) [1]. There are also other minor differences in the diagnostic criteria applied for prolapse; cystocele has been defined as when the bladder descends to any area below the PCL, and uterocervical prolapse and enterocele are when the cervix or small bowel are below the PCL .

6. Proposed protocol for upright open MRI evaluation of POP

Based on our literature search research, the protocol we propose for upright open MRI evaluation of women with prolapse and stress urinary incontinence is as follows. (1) All women complete a history that includes validated symptom scores for bladder, bowel, and prolapse-related symptoms. (2) Patients have a physical examination that follows IUGA/ICS guidelines [10]; this examination includes POPQ staging. (3) Patients complete a screening assessment tool to ensure there are no contraindications for magnetic resonance imaging. Some metals and surgical hardware are ferromagnetic and, therefore, are not acceptable with MRI. (4). Imaging is then conducted.

Our images are obtained currently using a 0.5 T scanner located at a dedicated research facility at the Centre for Hip Health at the University of British Columbia, Canada. Each patient's preparation includes ensuring a full bladder; hence, they are asked to refrain from voiding for 2 h before imaging. For standing images, intermittent pneumatic compression devices are applied to the legs. A T2-weighted sagittal image of the midline structures, including the symphysis, urethra, and coccyx, is acquired. Women then empty the bladder, and images in the supine, seated, and upright position are obtained. Current settings based on pilot studies indicate successful imaging is obtained with the following: TR/effective TE, 2500/16; echo train length, 32; bandwidth, 32 kHz; excitation, one; matrix size, 256 × 160; field of view, 0.5 (24 cm); section thickness, 5 mm, slice gap, 1. Sagittal images for mobility of the bladder neck and urethra can be obtained during straining [46].

7. Proposed clinical scenario for imaging

As an example of the benefits of this protocol, a 60-year-old multiparous woman presented with increasing urinary incontinence, constipation, a sensation of incomplete emptying, pelvic pressure, and pain. On pelvic examination (supine and inclined, at rest, and with Valsalva), no organ descent was detected. Conventional supine magnetic resonance imaging (MRI) did not identify pelvic organ prolapse (POP), but evaluation using upright open MRI diagnosed that organ prolapse involving the bladder occurred when standing. In **Figure 1** an example of anterior views of sagittal images showing gravity-induced quantification prolapse can be

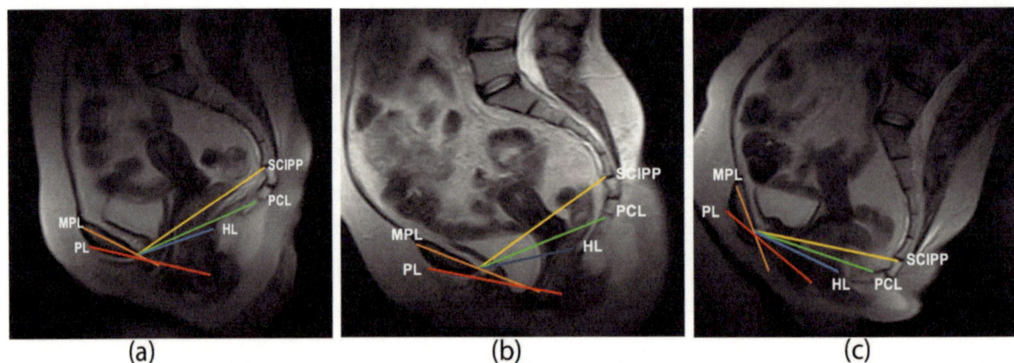

Figure 1. Anterior views of sagittal images show gravity-induced quantification prolapse. When a supine midsagittal single-shot fast SE image obtained at 0.5 T (panel A) and the corresponding image in standing (panel B) T2-weighted sagittal images of the female midline pelvic floor structures are compared, elongation of the bladder below the pubococcygeal reference line identifies significant prolapse when this patient is standing. A) Sagittal MRI image of female pelvis in the supine position, B) Sagittal MRI image of female pelvis in the standing position, C) Sagittal MRI image of female pelvis in the sitting position.

seen. When a supine midsagittal single-shot fast SE image obtained at 0.5 T (Panel A) and the corresponding image in standing (Panel B) also the corresponding image in sitting position (Panel C) T2-weighted sagittal images of the female midline pelvic floor structures are compared, elongation of the bladder below the pubococcygeal reference line identifies significant prolapse when this patient is standing.

8. 3D computer-generated images

An additional component for more comprehensive evaluation of POP is to generate 3D images. After mid-sagittal pelvic MRI scans are complete, the images are transmitted to a workstation for processing to generate 3D models. On average, 40 axial images were combined to generate each 3D model. The data were first segmented to anatomically major components, including bladder, urethra, vagina, uterus, rectum, obturator internus, and all three components of the levator ani (puborectalis, iliococcygeus, and coccygeus) using manual editing. Old reference 3D reconstruction is labor intensive and hence costly. However, the resulting images yield a huge amount of detailed information that simply cannot be obtained from 2D images. Moreover, use of mathematical modeling will be helpful in the future to assist in defining the relationships of organs and quantifying mobility and pressure gradients to resolve questions of continence and pelvic floor prolapse [47]. Further, advantages of 3D reconstruction include the additional data provided for patient–clinician interaction to enhance understanding, more comprehensive surgical planning, and to advance medical research, and education [46]. A three-dimensional model of the levator can be produced for living individuals and muscle volume calculated old reference.

The limitations include high cost and relative complexity of acquiring the initial images and the requirement for computer hardware and dedicated software [46]. Examples of the 3D imaging of the female pelvic floor can be seen in **Figure 2**.

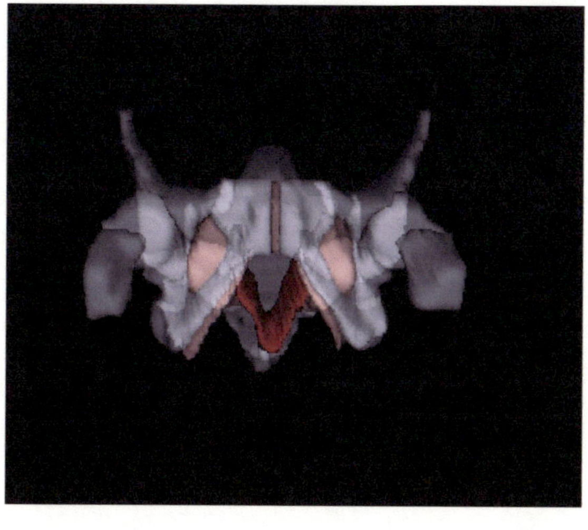

(A)

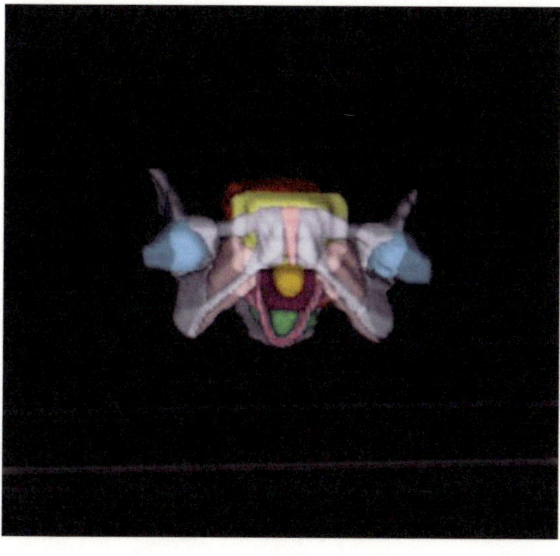

(B)

Figure 2. Three-dimensional imaging of the female pelvic floor: (A) anterior view of 3D pelvic floor model: (gray, pelvic bones), (pink, obturator internus m, piriformis m), (red, levator ani m). (B) Anterior view of 3D reconstruction of the whole female pelvis: (yellow, bladder, urethra), (red, uterus), (pink, vagina), (blue, rectum) as segmented from MRI images. A) Anterior view of 3D pelvic floor model as segmented from MRI images. B) Anterior view of 3D computer model of the whole female pelvis including supporting structures and organs.

9. Conclusions

Physicians should be aware that as upright open MRI becomes available this form of imaging will offer new levels of anatomic details relevant to a more accurate staging of POP and improved allocation to medical or surgical treatment. In POP, posture and gravity impact pelvic organ position, pelvic floor muscle integrity, degree of prolapse, and symptom severity. Importantly, while guidelines for clinical evaluation include recognition of the effects of posture, current imaging modalities are not always able to capture this aspect of prolapse. Ultrasound is a practical and widely available imaging modality. In patients who cannot bear MRI, CT may be beneficial as an alternate diagnostic process, but radiation is high. MRI provides multiplanar imaging and superior soft tissue contrast, permitting evaluation of the pelvic floor levator ani muscle in detail, but current imaging is limited to the supine position.

Reference lines related to bony anatomical landmarks allow prolapse to be quantified. 3D image reconstruction from 2D MRI images provides information beyond that acquired from 2D studies. Our upright open MRI imaging and 3D protocol makes comprehensive diagnostic imaging available that improves the accuracy of diagnosis and staging of POP.

Author details

Marwa Abdulaziz[1*], Lynn Stothers[2] and Andrew Macnab[2]

*Address all correspondence to: sonah_2008@hotmail.com

1 Department of Experimental Medicine, University of British Columbia, Vancouver, Canada

2 Department of Urological Sciences, University of British Columbia, Vancouver, Canada

References

[1] Haylen BT, Maher CF, Barber MD, Camargo S, Dandolu V, et al. An international urogynecological association (IUGA)/international continence society (ICS) joint report on the terminology for female pelvic organ prolapse (POP). International Urogynecology Journal. 2016;**27**(4):655-684

[2] Dietz HP. Pelvic floor ultrasound in prolapse: What's in it for the surgeon? International Urogynecology Journal. 2011;**22**(10):1221-1232

[3] Jeffcoate TN, Roberts H. Observations on stress incontinence of urine. American Journal of Obstetrics and Gynecology. 1952;**64**(4):721-738

[4] Kohorn EI, Scioscia AL, Jeanty P, Hobbins JC. Ultrasound cystourethrography by perineal scanning for the assessment of female stress urinary incontinence. Obstetrics and Gynecology. 1986;**68**(2):269-272

[5] Grischke EM, Dietz HP, Jeanty P, Schmidt W. A new study method: The perineal scan in obstetrics and gynecology. Ultraschall in der Medizin. 1986;**7**(4):154-161

[6] Dohke M, Mitchell DG, Vasavada SP. Fast magnetic resonance imaging of pelvic organ prolapse. Techniques in Urology. 2001;**7**(2):133-138

[7] Friedman B, Stothers L, Lazare D, Macnab A. Positional pelvic organ prolapse (POP) evaluation using open, weight-bearing magnetic resonance imaging (MRI). Canadian Urological Association Journal. 2015;**9**(5-6):197-200

[8] Nygaard I, Barber MD, Burgio KL, Kenton K, Meikle S, et al. Prevalence of symptomatic pelvic floor disorders in US women. JAMA. 2008;**300**(11):1311-1316. DOI: 10.1001/jama.300.11.1311

[9] Bo K, Finckenhagen HB. Vaginal palpation of pelvic floor muscle strength: Inter-test reproducibility and comparison between palpation and vaginal squeeze pressure. Acta Obstetricia et Gynecologica Scandinavica. 2001;**80**(10):883-887

[10] Barasinski C, Vendittelli F. Effect of the type of maternal pushing during the second stage of labour on obstetric and neonatal outcome: A multicentre randomised trial—The EOLE study protocol. BMJ Open 2016;**6**:e012290. DOI: 10.1136/bmjopen-2016- 012290

[11] Abrams P, Andersson KE, Birder L, Brubaker L, Cardozo L, et al. Fourth international consultation on incontinence recommendations of the international scientific committee: Evaluation and treatment of urinary incontinence, pelvic organ prolapse, and fecal incontinence. Neurourology and Urodynamics. 2010;**29**(1):213-240

[12] Dietz HP, Lanzarone V. Levator trauma after vaginal delivery. Obstetrics and Gynecology. 2005;**106**(4):707-712

[13] Dietz HP, Steensma AB. The prevalence of major abnormalities of the levator ani in urogynaecological patients. BJOG : An International Journal of Obstetrics and Gynaecology. 2006;**113**(2):225-230

[14] DeLancey JOL, Morgan DM, Fenner DE, Kearney R, Guire K, et al. Comparison of levator ani muscle defects and function in women with and without pelvic organ prolapse. Obstetrics and Gynecology. 2007;**109**(2 Pt 1):295-302

[15] Shek KL, Dietz HP. Intrapartum risk factors for levator trauma. BJOG : An International Journal of Obstetrics and Gynaecology. 2010;**117**(12):1485-1492

[16] Shek KL, Chantarasorn V, Langer S, Phipps H, Dietz HP. Does the Epi-no birth trainer reduce levator trauma? A randomised controlled trial. International Urogynecology Journal. 2011;**22**(12):1521-1528

[17] Dietz HP, Gillespie AV, Phadke P. Avulsion of the pubovisceral muscle associated with large vaginal tear after normal vaginal delivery at term. The Australian & New Zealand Journal of Obstetrics & Gynaecology. 2007;**47**(4):341-344

[18] Dietz HP, Shek KL, Daly O, Korda A. Can levator avulsion be repaired surgically? A prospective surgical pilot study. International Urogynecology Journal. 2013;**24**(6):1011-1015

[19] Dietz HP. Pelvic floor ultrasound: A review. American Journal of Obstetrics and Gynecology. 2010;**202**(4):321-334

[20] Athanasiou S, Chaliha C, Toozs-Hobson P, Salvatore S, Khullar V, Cardozo L. Direct imaging of the pelvic floor muscles using two-dimensional ultrasound: A comparison of women with urogenital prolapse versus controls. BJOG: An International Journal of Obstetrics and Gynaecology. 2007;**114**(7):882-888

[21] Tunn R, Paris S, Taupitz M, Hamm B, Fischer W. MR imaging in posthysterectomy vaginal prolapse. International Urogynecology Journal and Pelvic Floor Dysfunction. 2000; **11**(2):87-92

[22] Pannu HK. Magnetic resonance imaging of pelvic organ prolapse. Abdominal Imaging. 2002;**27**(6):660-673

[23] Reiner CS, Weishaupt D. Dynamic pelvic floor imaging: MRI techniques and imaging parameters. Abdominal Imaging. 2013;**38**(5):903-911

[24] Bo K, Finckenhagen HB. Is there any difference in measurement of pelvic floor muscle strength in supine and standing position? Acta Obstetricia et Gynecologica Scandinavica. 2003;**82**(12):1120-1124

[25] Parkkinen A, Karjalainen E, Vartiainen M, Penttinen J. Physiotherapy for female stress urinary incontinence: Individual therapy at the outpatient clinic versus home-based pelvic floor training: A 5-year follow-up study. Neurourology and Urodynamics. 2004; **23**(7):643-648

[26] Hendrix SL, Clark A, Nygaard I, Aragaki A, Barnabei V, McTiernan A. Pelvic organ prolapse in the Women's Health Initiative: Gravity and gravidity. American Journal of Obstetrics and Gynecology. 2002;**186**(6):1160-1166

[27] Dietz HP, Clarke B. The influence of posture on perineal ultrasound imaging parameters. International Urogynecology Journal and Pelvic Floor Dysfunction. 2001;**12**(2):104-106

[28] Bertschinger KM, Hetzer FH, Roos JE, Treiber K, Marincek B, Hilfiker PR. Dynamic MR imaging of the pelvic floor performed with patient sitting in an open-magnet unit versus with patient supine in a closed-magnet unit. Radiology. 2002;**223**(2):501-508

[29] Flusberg M, Sahni VA, Erturk SM, Mortele KJ. Dynamic MR defecography: Assessment of the usefulness of the defecation phase. AJR. American Journal of Roentgenology. 2011; **196**(4):W394-W399

[30] Dietz HP. Ultrasound imaging of the pelvic floor. Part I: Two-dimensional aspects. Ultrasound in Obstetrics & Gynecology. 2004;**23**(1):80-92

[31] Mouritsen L, Bernstein I. Vaginal ultrasonography: A diagnostic tool for urethral diverticulum. Acta Obstetricia et Gynecologica Scandinavica. 1996;**75**(2):188-190

[32] Siegel CL, Middleton WD, Teefey SA, Wainstein MA, McDougall EM, Klutke CG. Sonography of the female urethra. AJR. American Journal of Roentgenology. 1998; **170**(5):1269-1274

[33] Pannu HK, Genadry R, Kaufman HS, Fishman EK. Computed tomography evaluation of pelvic organ prolapse. Techniques and applications. Journal of Computer Assisted Tomography. 2003;**27**(5):779-785

[34] Kaufman HS, Buller JL, Thimpson RJ, Pannu HK, DeMeester SL, et al. Dynamic pelvic magnetic resonance imaging and cystocolpoproctography alter surgical management of pelvic floor disorders. Diseases of the Colon and Rectum. 2001;**44**(11):1575-1583. discussion 1583-4

[35] Comiter CV, Vasavada SP, Barbaric ZL, Gousse AE, Raz S. Grading pelvic prolapse and pelvic floor relaxation using dynamic magnetic resonance imaging. Urology. 1999; **54**(3):454-457

[36] Pizzoferrato AC, Nyangoh Timoh K, Fritel X, Zareski E, Bader G, Fauconnier A. Dynamic magnetic resonance imaging and pelvic floor disorders: How and when? European Journal of Obstetrics, Gynecology, and Reproductive Biology. 2014;**181**:259-266

[37] Fauconnier A, Zareski E, Abichedid J, Bader G, Falissard B, Fritel X. Dynamic magnetic resonance imaging for grading pelvic organ prolapse according to the international continence society classification: Which line should be used? Neurourology and Urodynamics. 2008;**27**(3):191-197

[38] Woodfield CA, Hampton BS, Sung V, Brody JM. Magnetic resonance imaging of pelvic organ prolapse: Comparing pubococcygeal and midpubic lines with clinical staging. International Urogynecology Journal and Pelvic Floor Dysfunction. 2009;**20**(6):695-701

[39] Fritel X, Fauconnier A, Bader G, Cosson M, Debodinance P, et al. Diagnosis and management of adult female stress urinary incontinence: Guidelines for clinical practice from the French College of Gynaecologists and Obstetricians. European Journal of Obstetrics, Gynecology, and Reproductive Biology. 2010;**151**(1):14-19

[40] Law PA, Danin JC, Lamb GM, Regan L, Darzi A, Gedroyc WM. Dynamic imaging of the pelvic floor using an open-configuration magnetic resonance scanner. Journal of Magnetic Resonance Imaging. 2001;**13**(6):923-929

[41] Orno AK, Dietz HP. Levator co-activation is a significant confounder of pelvic organ descent on Valsalva maneuver. Ultrasound in Obstetrics & Gynecology. 2007;**30**(3):346-350

[42] Dvorkin LS, Hetzer F, Scott SM, Williams NS, Gedroyc W, Lunniss PJ. Open-magnet MR defaecography compared with evacuation proctography in the diagnosis and management of patients with rectal intussusception. Colorectal Disease. 2004;**6**(1):45-53

[43] Roos JE, Weishaupt D, Wildermuth S, Willmann JK, Marincek B, Hilfiker PR. Experience of 4 years with open MR defecography: Pictorial review of anorectal anatomy and disease. Radiographics. 2002;**22**(4):817-832

[44] Broekhuis SR, Fütterer JJ, Barentsz JO, Vierhout ME, Kluivers KB. A systematic review of clinical studies on dynamic magnetic resonance imaging of pelvic organ prolapse: The use of reference lines and anatomical landmarks. International Urogynecology Journal and Pelvic Floor Dysfunction. 2009;**20**(6):721-729

[45] Singh K, Reid WM, Berger LA. Assessment and grading of pelvic organ prolapse by use of dynamic magnetic resonance imaging. American Journal of Obstetrics and Gynecology. 2001;**185**(1):71-77

[46] Abdulaziz M, Deegan EG, Kavanagh A, Stothers L, Pugash D, Macnab A. Advances in basic science methodologies for clinical diagnosis in female stress urinary incontinence. Canadian Urological Association Journal. 2017;**11**(6Suppl2):S117-S120

[47] Otcenasek M, Krofta L, Baca V, Grill R, Kucera E, et al. Bilateral avulsion of the puborectal muscle: Magnetic resonance imaging-based three-dimensional reconstruction and comparison with a model of a healthy nulliparous woman. Ultrasound in Obstetrics & Gynecology. 2007;**29**(6):692-696

Chapter 4

Synthetic Materials Used in the Surgical Treatment of Pelvic Organ Prolapse: Problems of Currently Used Material and Designing the Ideal Material

Naşide Mangir, Christopher R. Chapple and
Sheila MacNeil

Additional information is available at the end of the chapter

http://dx.doi.org/10.5772/intechopen.76671

Abstract

Synthetic materials have long been used to provide structural support when surgically repairing pelvic organ prolapse (POP). The most widely used synthetic material is a mesh made of polypropylene (PPL). The use of mesh is intended to improve cure rates and prevent recurrences after POP surgery – however as more mesh materials have been implanted, it has become apparent that serious complications can occur in up to 30% of women, particularly when the mesh is implanted transvaginally. Over the years many different mesh kits have been marketed and used in the treatment of POP however polypropylene mesh was never designed or tested for use in pelvic floor. Instead it was approved for clinical use based on its biocompatibility and success in abdominal hernia repairs. It is now known that PPL meshes are neither compliant with the mechanical forces in the pelvic floor nor do they integrate well into paravaginal tissues. Better materials developed specifically for use in pelvic floor are urgently needed. The aim of this chapter is to define the requirements of an ideal mesh in terms of its material properties and to summarize the ongoing research on developing the next generation pelvic floor repair materials.

Keywords: pelvic organ prolapse, mesh, polypropylene, implant material, biomechanical properties

1. Introduction

Pelvic organ prolapse (POP) is the descent of one or more of the anterior vaginal wall, posterior vaginal wall, the uterus (cervix) or the apex of the vagina (after hysterectomy) which

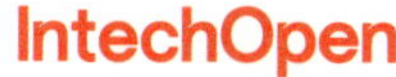

correlates with patients' symptoms [1]. Prolapse of the anterior vaginal wall (or a cystocele) is the most common type of POP followed by a uterine or vault prolapse and rectal prolapse [2], although they coexist in most patients presenting with symptomatic POP.

Some degree of POP is seen in up to 30–76% of women who have their routine gynaecological examinations [3]. Most of these will be early stage/mild prolapses and cause no symptoms [4]. Although only 3–6% of these cases will have any symptoms, the lifetime risk of a women in the general population undergoing a POP surgery has been reported to be 20% (excluding hysterectomy cases) [3]. As the population ages the prevalence of POP is estimated to increase substantially by 46% between 2010 and 2050 [5].

Reconstructive surgery to improve positioning of the pelvic organs or to restore the supporting structures is often necessary in symptomatic cases and the use of a graft material is often needed to reinforce weakened tissues. The most commonly used material is a surgical mesh made of polypropylene (PPL) which has long been used successfully to treat hernias. Although mesh augmented POP repair procedures have higher anatomical success rates compared to no-mesh, the functional and quality of life outcomes are not as good [6] and severe complications with life changing consequences can occur in up to 10–30% of cases [7]. Complications associated with the use of vaginal mesh are now reported widely in the media together with many litigations against physicians and manufacturers leading to the withdrawal of several mesh products from the USA market [8]. In the UK there are now 800 compensation claims made against the NHS in relation to vaginal mesh related complications [9]. In 2008 and 2011 the Food and Drug Administration (FDA) of United States of America released two public health warnings related to mesh complications [10] which was followed by statements from Medicines and Healthcare products Regulatory Agency (MHRA) in United Kingdom [11] and the European Commission [12]. Consequently transvaginal meshes were re-classified from being class II (a moderate risk device) to class III (a high risk device) making pre-market approval necessary before new devices could be marketed [13]. As a consequence the relative number of mesh augmented transvaginal POP repair procedures decreased sharply from 27 to 2%, among all other types of POP surgeries [14]. The number of mesh sling surgeries for treatment of stress urinary incontinence has also decreased [15].

Factors affecting occurrence of mesh related complications can broadly be classified as factors related to the material itself and factors related to the application of the material [16]. Material properties involve the composition of the polymer used, total bulk of the material used and its biocompatibility, mechanical properties and ultrastructure such as pore size and knit pattern. Factors related to the application of the material are the surgical technique used, the route of implantation [transvaginal vs. transabdominal], surgeon's experience and patient related factors [obesity, smoking status, etc.].

In this chapter we will first explore the evolvement of the surgical mesh as a material used in abdominal hernia repair together with the modifications made to the surgical technique of implantation to improve patient outcomes. We then move on to define the mechanical and biological properties of the female pelvic floor to determine the design requirements of the ideal pelvic floor repair material. Finally we will look at the current approaches to develop novel materials using mainly biomaterials and tissue engineering techniques with reference to some of the work from our own group.

2. The use of materials in pelvic surgery

In pelvic organ prolapse surgeries, prosthetic materials are either needed to reinforce the surgical repair site in anterior and posterior vaginal wall defect repairs or to suspend the prolapsed uterus or vaginal vault in sacrocolpopexy operations [17]. Surgeries performed for stress urinary incontinence use this material under the urethra as a sling.

The ideal prosthetic material is desired to provide a durable structural support without causing significant complications such as pain, compromise in vaginal capacity or sexual functions. A wide variety of synthetic and biological materials have been used over the years as prosthetics however the perfect material is still to be developed.

Biological materials are mostly in the form of biological grafts from the patient's own tissues from abdomen (rectus fascia) or thigh (fascia lata). These autologous fascia have long been used as a sling in the treatment of stress urinary incontinence [18]. The obvious limitation of using an autologous fascia is increased perioperative morbidity, donor site morbidity and lack of availability of enough material in some patients who require repeated procedures or have large areas of fascia defect. Using natural fascia from allogeneic (e.g. cadaveric) or xenogeneic (e.g. bovine dermis) sources has also been used over the years but these carry a small risk of prion and Human Immunodeficiency Virus transmission. Also the decellularization, sterilization and other processing methods are known to adversely influence the biomechanical properties of the fascia [19]. The clinical efficacy of biological implants are still controversial with some studies showing high anatomical and functional failure rates [20, 21] whereas others report results comparable to mesh repairs in less severe cases of POP [22].

A basic understanding of the material properties of the available grafts and the physiological requirements of the site of implantation is required to select the best material for a specific application.

3. Evolvement of the polypropylene mesh as a material

The concept of using a prosthetic material to reinforce a fascial defect was first developed to treat hernias. Theodore Billroth (1829–1894) stated that "If we could artificially produce tissues of the density and toughness of fascia and tendon the secret of the radical cure of hernia would be discovered" Czerny [23]. The first mesh material was made of metal. In 1902 silver filigrees were used to treat difficult to treat hernias [24]. The silver wires and other metals (tantalum and stainless steel) were used until recently [25] with reasonable success rates to treat large hernia defects however they were eventually abandoned due to their association with excessive abdominal stiffness, sinus tract formation, metal failure (corrosion and fragmentation) and patient discomfort.

Following the plastics revolution in 20th century and the advancements in polymer science many diagnostic and therapeutic medical and surgical instruments made of plastic became available. Plastics had obvious advantages over metals in soft tissue reconstruction with their ductility, lightweight and handleability [26]. Among the plastics used, polypropylene (PPL) possessed favorable physical properties such as high tensile strength with easy handleability. It could be made into a monofilament, have a high softening temperature (260°F), non wettable and resistant to chemicals. Usher first manufactured and experimentally tested first plastic mesh made of polypropylene [27]. The initial experimental data in dogs with knitted PPL confirmed that it allowed tissue ingrowth in between its fibers, it was strong with excellent tensile properties and it was resistant to infections when compared to other plastics.

The use of synthetic mesh has revolutionized hernia repair surgeries reducing the recurrence rates by 2–3 fold compared to traditional suture repairs [28]. However looking retrospectively it appears that PPL was far from being complication-free when first introduced into abdominal hernia repairs. Over the years, both the surgical implantation site and the material properties of the PPL have been modified to reduce the complication rates of mesh augmented abdominal hernia repair surgeries. A brief revision of the improvements made to the surgical technique and material characteristics over many years can provide a better understanding of the current clinical problem related to vaginal mesh products.

The initial plastic mesh was prepared from a monofilament 8 mils in diameter (200 μm), 42 × 40 per inch thread count by a simple taffeta weave. This mesh was then autoclaved and cut into desired patterns before implantation [33]. On the other hand, the modern surgical mesh constructed from a knitted polypropylene has smaller pores with an area density of 90–95 g/m^2. These heavy-weight, first generation meshes are now known to cause a vigorous foreign body reaction and resulting dense scar tissue leading to a loss of the compliance of the abdominal wall [34].

Over the next few years heavy weight meshes were replaced by medium to light weight meshes that reduced the bulk of the foreign material leading to less inflammation, foreign body reaction, fibrosis and the associated pain sensation [34]. Also the pore sizes were made larger (macroporous). A study demonstrated that the bulk density of PPL (Prolene®) mesh could be reduced down to 25% of its original weight without significantly compromising its efficacy with reduced major and minor complications [35]. Also clinical studies comparing

1902 [24]	First prosthetic mesh (silver filigrees) to be routinely used to treat difficult to treat hernias.
1940 [29]	Tantalum gauze fabric introduced
1948 [30]	Formation of a darn using a Nylon suture for inguinal hernia repair.
1963	Francis Usher (1908–1980) introduced first woven, plastic mesh made of polypropylene for hernia repair.
1995 [31]	Ulmsten and Petros described the Integral theory of stress urinary continence and performed the first intravaginal mesh-sling surgery
1996*	PPL (Marlex®) received FDA clearance for SUI.
1998*	First lightweight PPL mesh introduced.
2002*	First mesh product for POP (Gyneacare®).
2004*	First 'mesh kit' (Apogee®, Perigee®) cleared by FDA for POP.

*Reviewed in Dällenbach [32].

Table 1. Milestones in the development of surgical mesh materials and their use in pelvic floor disorders.

http://dx.doi.org/10.5772/intechopen.76671

heavy and light-weight mesh materials implanted for inguinal hernia repairs demonstrated less pain and less sensation of a foreign material with lighter meshes [36]. Thus the polypropylene mesh evolved over the years from a heavy weight, small pore sized mesh to a light-weight, and large pore sized mesh material.

Efforts to make further improvements to the current surgical mesh are still ongoing. One strategy to modify the geometry/knitting pattern of PPL to make it mechanically more compliant with the pelvic floor [37]. Another strategy is enhancing the biocompatibility of PPL by coating it with more biocompatible materials to obtain a more favorable tissue response. An extracellular matrix coated PPL when implanted in rats demonstrated an inflammatory response that is more reflective of a tissue remodeling type rather than a fibrotic one [38]. There has also been research on degradable and hybrid degradable/nondegradable mesh materials. The main idea behind a degradable mesh was that it would be absorbed after a period of time by which time the patients' own tissues would have recovered and this would avoid the long term complications of permanent mesh like infection and fistula formation. Nevertheless polypropylene is still the most widely used polymer in mesh products used clinically at the time of writing.

4. Modifications to the surgical technique to improve outcomes of mesh-augmented hernia repairs

In parallel to improvements made to the material, modifications to the surgical technique were also made to reduce side effects and recurrences. Advances in both inguinal and abdominal hernia repair techniques can be observed mainly led by Usher and Rives [39]. Usher has also made contributions to developing the technique of hernia repair, mainly he introduced the concept of buttressing a sutured repair instead of bridging the gap with a mesh. On other words the mesh would not only just fit in the hole but be 2–3 cm larger to underlap with the underlying tissues.

We will only review the improvements made to the surgical approach to incisional hernia repair in the abdominal wall, where we feel it is relevant to the pelvic floor repair. The abdominal hernia repair technique evolved from an 'inlay technique' where the mesh is placed in-between the edges of the fascia defect to an 'onlay technique' where the mesh was placed on top of the repaired fascia defect in a tension-free manner. To further reduce the complications of mesh augmented repairs, a 'sublay (retrorectus) technique' was introduced where the mesh was placed underneath a well vascularized, thick muscle tissue (the rectus abdominis muscle) in-between two fascial layers (**Figure 1**). Proximity to a well vascularized wound bed is arguably a key factor in the success of this technique [40]. Additionally in the sublay technique, as opposed to inlay and onlay, mesh had less contact with subcutaneous tissues that prevented transmission of the infection from subcutaneous tissues to the mesh as it lies quite deep in the abdominal wall [41]. Abdominal hernias are heterogeneous with regards to why they occur and how extensive they are. No single technique is suitable or feasible for all types of hernias and different methods of repair may be indicated for specific defects and locations. Nevertheless the sublay technique appears to be superior to other techniques particularly in difficult to treat wound beds (for example poorly vascularized or repeatedly operated wounds) [42, 43].

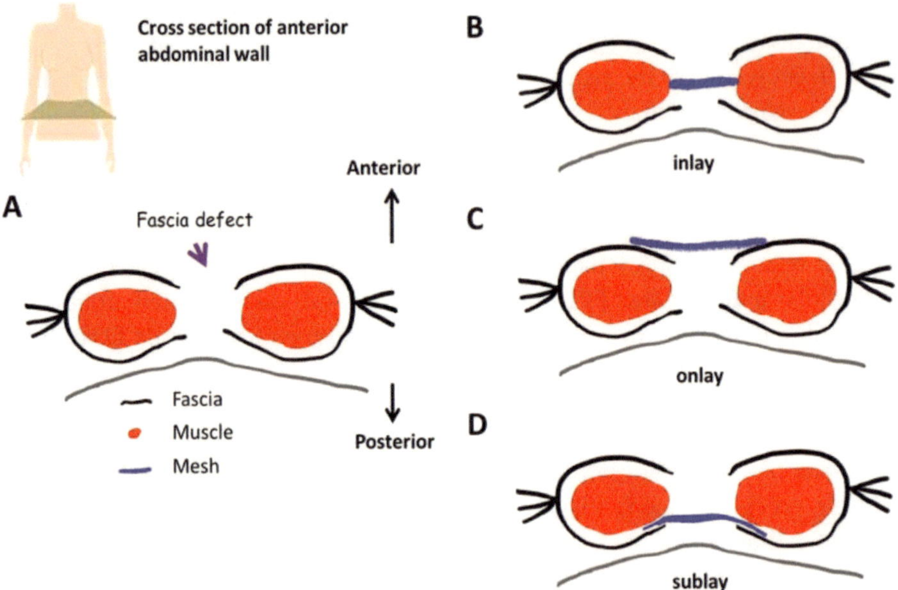

Figure 1. Graphical demonstration of surgical implantation sites of mesh material in relation to muscle and fascia in abdominal hernia repairs. (A) A cross section of anterior abdominal wall with a fascia defect causing hernia can be seen with muscle (red), fascia (black) and mesh (blue) labeled in different colors. (B) Inlay mesh implantation to fit in the gap created by the fascia and muscle defect. This method was largely abandoned due to high recurrence rates. (C) Onlay placement of mesh material to overlie and reinforce the fascia and muscle defect. (D) In the sublay technique mesh material is placed on a well vascularized wound bed underneath the muscle and it is also covered by two fascial layers. This technique is considered the current gold standard with less complication and high success rates.

5. The failure of PPL in the pelvic floor

The first use of polypropylene in the pelvic floor was based on the integral theory [44]. The integral theory of female stress urinary incontinence stated that the pubourethral ligament in women creates a physiologic 'backboard' by fixing the mid-urethra to the pubic bone and that the laxity of this ligament results in the loss of the backboard inhibiting the urethral coaptation during times of increased intra-abdominal pressure that results in urinary incontinence. The synthetic midurethral slings (MUS) based on the integral theory came as a minimally invasive treatment modality with very high success rates. The initial description of the methodology used plastic tapes with the patient under local anesthesia [31]. The high initial success rates of the minimally invasive, relatively easy to perform MUS operations soon led to the use of the PPL mesh for transvaginal repair of pelvic organ prolapse.

The POP occurs as a result of loss of support at three levels in the pelvis. Level I cardinal-uterosacral ligaments providing apical support, level II arcus tendineus fascia pelvis supporting middle part of vagina laterally and level III urogenital diaphragm and perineal body supporting lower part of the vagina [45]. The contribution of each of these structures to occurrence of prolapse as we see it in the clinic, is not well defined. A recent work, for example, suggests that lack of vaginal apical support was a significant contributor to the occurrence of anterior compartment prolapse and that correcting the apical descent when treating cystoceles would reduce re-operation rates [46]. Thus the exact pathophysiology of POP, its correlations with clinical presentations and the theoretical basis of surgical techniques performed to treat POP are not well described. Nevertheless most of POP repair procedures are performed via a vaginal route (transvaginally) [47] either by placing the mesh directly on to the native tissue repair or suturing it to a strong ligament such as the sacrospinous ligament or arcus tendinous fascia pelvis [17]. Regardless of at what level the defect is and what the mesh restores, the transvaginal POP repair is more reflective of an onlay technique (mesh onlay repair) which did not work very well in the abdomen arguably due to being prone to be colonized by skin microbial flora as it lies very close to the skin [48]. Additionally, the mesh is not placed on a well vascularized wound bed in mesh onlay vaginal repairs. This can have particular importance in the postmenopausal women undergoing these operations as they already have poorly oestrogenised tissues.

In addition to the limitations related to the surgical technique of implantation, the PPL mesh also has some inherent characteristics that make it unsuitable for use in pelvic floor. Recent animal studies in sheep confirmed a site specific response to implanted PPL mesh, where a 5 × 5 cm piece of PPL mesh led to contraction and erosion in 3 out of 10 sheep in 12 months when implanted vaginally in contrast to no erosions in abdominal implantations [49]. The animal studies also showed that the host response to the PPL initiated by macrophages in the mesh-tissue interface was mainly an M1 (proinflammatory) response, instead of an M2 (remodeling) response, characterized by secretion of matrix metalloproteinases and pro-inflammatory cytokines leading to a vigorous foreign body reaction [50]. An M2 response is favorable for tissue integration while an M1 dominated response is now thought to explain the pain associated with mesh and mesh exposure. Clinical data obtained from women who underwent mesh excision due to severe pain or mesh exposure also confirmed that there was an M1 predominant macrophage response observed in the histological sections of the mesh-vagina explants [51]. Essentially a high M1 response indicates persistent inflammation. Thus there is a site-specific response to PPL mesh and the failure of PPL in the pelvic floor is partially due to the unfavorable mesh-tissue interaction leading to poor tissue integration.

In conclusion the use of mesh evolved over many years from an initial metal wire mesh to the monofilament, macroporous PPL mesh used in contemporary practice. Together with the improvements made in the surgical implantation technique mesh augmented surgical repairs now have very reasonable success rates in abdominal hernia surgeries. Although some of these improvements made to the material have been translated to the pelvic floor, we know that the same material when implanted vaginally to treat POP has resulted in unacceptably high complication rates.

This can be partially explained by factors related to the current surgical technique. The standard surgical technique, particularly those of transvaginal POP repairs, may need further improvements which will clearly require a better understanding of the pathophysiology of POP in women. Another important aspect is related to the pre and postoperative factors. It is now recognized that mesh augmented pelvic floor repair procedures, although conducted as minimally invasive day case procedures, involve placement of a permanent implant into the patients' body making post implantation surveillance necessary [12, 16]. Also factors related to patient selection, especially when the patients have co-morbidities such as diabetes and obesity, are known to influence postoperative outcomes. Surgeons' experience is another potentially important factor in the mesh implant procedures. Several recent consensus reports on how to control vaginal mesh related complications are now emphasizing that only surgeons/centers with subspecialist experience on implantation and postoperative management of patients with stress urinary incontinence and pelvic organ prolapse should undertake these procedures. Also the implementation of national mesh registries, thus not relying solely on the manufacturers to report mesh related adverse event and mandatory post-implantation surveillance systems are recommended.

6. Designing synthetic materials to be used in pelvic floor reconstruction

The PPL vaginal meshes in current clinical use were never designed or tested specifically for use in pelvic floor. Instead they were cleared in regulatory terms based on their biocompatibility and the similarity of their textile properties to the existing abdominal hernia products via a 510(k) loophole. In other words, PPL mesh was used in pelvic floor based on an assumption that if it worked well in the abdomen to reinforce hernia repairs it would work equally well to support vaginal prolapse repairs. It is now being recognized that this approach was inherently flawed as the microbial flora, pH, vascular supply and physiological mechanical requirements of the pelvic floor are different from that of the abdomen.

Novel synthetic materials that are mechanically compatible with the requirements of the pelvic floor and that can effectively integrate into host tissues after implantation can be designed by using biomaterials and tissue engineering techniques. This requires an in depth understanding of the mechanical and biochemical properties of the pelvic floor. This section will review the available evidence on the biomechanics of the pelvic floor with a view to defining the design requirements for pelvic floor tissue engineering.

6.1. Basic definitions in biomechanics

The pelvic floor is the hammock-like structure made up of skeletal and smooth muscles surrounded by connective tissues and attached to pelvic bones. Its' main function is to counteract the forces generated by gravity and intra-abdominal pressure. When studying bioengineering of the pelvic floor we need to consider its biological constitution in relation to the mechanical forces acting on it. Namely, any material used to support the pelvic floor needs to have defined characteristics of material deformation and load bearing as well as how it contributes to tissue remodeling once it is implanted in to the body. It is important that clinicians/surgeons have a basic understanding of biomechanical principles so that they can define the biomechanics of the tissue to be replaced and select the best material to meet the specific needs.

Briefly, when a force is applied to a material it cause a change in size or shape of the material (deformation). This is most commonly expressed in a stress-strain curve from a uniaxial tensile test (**Figure 2**). This test gives an idea about the maximum forces needed to break the material (ultimate tensile strength) and the point where plastic deformation starts (yield strength). These parameters need to be considered together with the requirements of the site of implantation when designing an implant material.

6.2. Defining the mechanical characteristics of the native human pelvic floor

Our knowledge on the mechanical properties of the female pelvic floor mainly comes from mechanical testing of samples from the pelvic floor from human and animal samples. The availability of human samples for mechanical testing is often limited due to challenges and ethical concerns related to obtaining large tissue samples. Whole pelvic floor samples of animals that contain all the muscles and the connective tissues of the pelvic floor (e.g. 'vaginal supportive tissue complex') have been obtained from rats demonstrating that the ultimate failure in the testing protocol was due to a failure of paravaginal attachments [52]. Samples that only contain the connective tissues (e.g. fascia) have also been tested [53]. Disruption in the fascial structures is thought to be the main mechanism by which pelvic organ prolapse occurs [52].

Another factor limiting our ability to have robust definitions of mechanical properties of pelvic floor structures is the lack of standardized mechanical testing protocols for biological tissue samples. To obtain reproducible results when mechanically testing biological samples their unique organization, composition and *in vivo* functions need to be adopted to the mechanical testing protocols. Currently mechanical testing of samples from animal or human pelvic floor can mainly be tested by uniaxial and biaxial tensile testing. In uniaxial testing, the tissue to be tested is placed between two clamps (clamp-to-clamp testing) and a load is applied to the sample in one direction while observing for elongation/strain. Uniaxial testing is most commonly performed in these studies and it gives more reproducible results.

From a biomechanical point of view, the pelvic floor is a complex structure composed of active (e.g. muscles) and passive soft tissue (e.g. fascia) components attached to the pelvic bones all

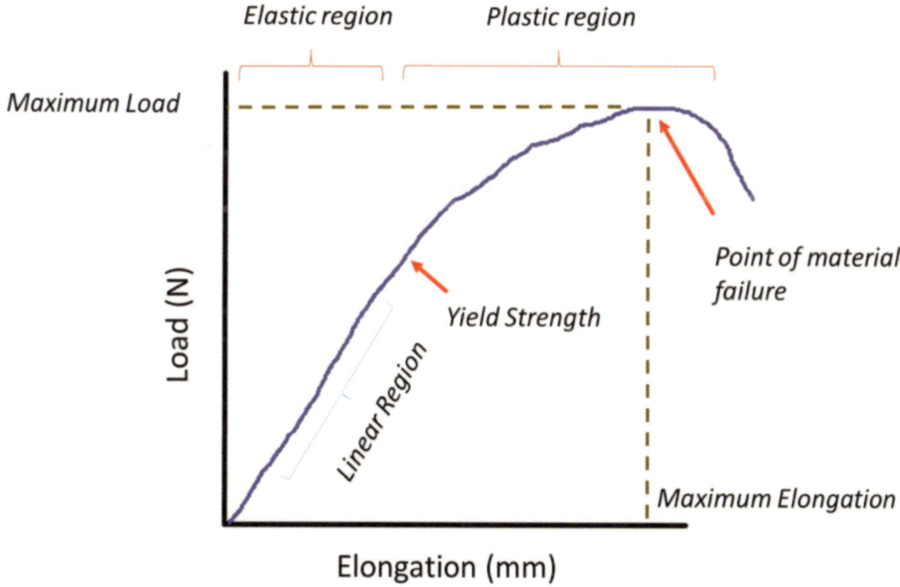

Figure 2. Defining the basic mechanical properties of a material by uniaxial mechanical testing. The 'maximum load' is the maximum amount of stress that a material can bear before it fails. The 'maximum elongation' is the maximum strain a material can achieve before it fails. The 'yield strength' is where irreversible deformation to the material starts.

contributing to the mechanical strength [54]. Computational models have the potential to mathematically combine all the complex anatomical, mechanical and biochemical data pertinent to pelvic floor to create computational models predicting the biomechanical behavior of the female pelvic floor in health and disease. Anatomical models demonstrating detailed 3D anatomy of the pelvic floor can now be reliably produced thanks to magnetic resonance imaging [55]. The remaining considerable challenge seems to be integrating the functionality of the muscles and other soft tissues into these models. The hope they offer is that once an accurate biomechanical model is created, population based data can be applied to these models before they are used clinically to predict individual patient/disease outcomes.

6.3. Biological requirements of pelvic floor

Early materials implanted into the human body were designed to have appropriate physical properties to match tissues at the site of implantation and to be made of materials which would have minimal toxicity. These materials were biologically 'inert' which ensured a minimal immune response to the foreign material. Although the consideration of the predicted immune response to an implanted material is still conceptually valid, there is a shift of paradigm about the inertness of a biomaterial. The next generation of biomaterials were purposefully designed to be bioactive to achieve a desired reaction post-implantation (e.g. antibiotic or extracellular matrix coated materials). Additionally the degradation times of the materials started to be finely tuned with advancements in resorbable biomaterials. The main advantage of using a degradable material would be that the foreign material would eventually be degraded after guiding the host to achieve a desired tissue regeneration (e.g. absorbable sutures commonly used in surgery).

The polypropylene material commonly used is traditionally considered 'inert'. Although PPL completely degrades over many years, its' inertness is now questioned after repeated demonstrations of surface degradation on the PPL fibers [56, 57]. The most common complication of surgical implantation of the mesh is spontaneous pain, occurring in 32.5% patients (pain during sexual intercourse 14.7%) [58]. The mechanisms leading to this pain are complex, probably involving infection, nerve and muscle injury and mesh contraction [59]. It has been demonstrated in mesh samples explanted from patients that PPL can actually degrade *in vivo* as early as 18 months after implantation [56]. This PPL polymer can breakdown in response to high temperature, UV light and oxidation [57].

Another important point to consider is the tissue specific immune response to the implanted biomaterial. The host immune system, mainly affected by tissue macrophages, initiate a cascade of events as soon as the material is implanted in the body. These reactions mainly take place at the material-tissue interface meaning that the surface structure and chemistry can potentially influence the initial macrophage response to the implanted material. Modifications of the surface properties of materials have been investigated as a potential strategy to shift the macrophage polarization towards a constructive remodeling type (M2) of reaction instead of a pro-inflammatory (M1) type. A well described pathway leading to biomaterial failure in the long term is development of a foreign body reaction leading to encapsulation of the material isolating it from the surrounding tissues. A foreign body reaction is a result of chronic M1 predominated inflammatory reaction. It has been demonstrated that synthetic materials when designed with a highly porous structure elicit less chronic inflammation leading to encapsulation [60, 61].

It is now widely accepted that the failure of PPL in pelvic floor is due to its mechanical incompatibility and the unfavorable mesh-tissue interaction leading to poor tissue integration. Essentially the PPL mesh is too strong and not elastic enough to be used in the pelvic floor [62, 63]. Additionally, animal studies have confirmed that the host response to the PPL initiated by macrophages in the mesh-tissue interface is mainly an M1 (proinflammatory) response, instead of an M2 (remodeling) response, characterized by secretion of matrix metalloproteinases and pro-inflammatory cytokines leading to a vigorous and persistent foreign body reaction [50]. Thus PPL is biologically and mechanically not the best material for pelvic floor repair. A recent European consensus report acknowledged the need for more research into more acceptable materials for use in the pelvic floor [12].

In conclusion when designing a material for use in the pelvic floor, the design characteristics should be optimized to consider its biodegradation and immunological response to it. When defining degradability of a material *in vivo* degradation characteristics and degradation products need to be defined. In case of non-degradable materials the chemical and mechanical changes to the material over many years need to be considered. Irrespective of this the host response to the material needs to be investigated in terms of both the acute and the longer term immunological response to the material. Finally its resistance to infection needs to be considered-this is often a combination of the material and its method of implantation.

7. Tissue engineering approaches to design novel materials to be used in pelvic floor repair

Tissue engineering and regenerative medicine can meet the clinical need in this area by either constructing biodegradable scaffolds that the host cells and tissues can use to remodel or directly by constructing a cell-tissue construct for implantation.

Compared to tissue engineering of other organs, such as bone and blood vessels, the area of pelvic floor tissue engineering is newly developing necessitating a better understanding of pelvic floor anatomy, physiology and mechanics. The first tissue engineered approach to construct an autologous fascia equivalent for POP repair was reported in 2010. In this study human vaginal fibroblasts were seeded on a PLGA knitted mesh before implantation into nude mice for 12 weeks and a well-organized new fascia with a high collagen I/III ratio was demonstrated [64]. A stronger tissue engineered material was also constructed from knitted silk mesh seeded with adipose derived MSCs in 2013 [65]. In 2013 comparative studies evaluated novel synthetic materials such as polyetheretherketone and polyamide as alternative materials to the PPL [66]. A gelatin-coated polyamide knit mesh seeded with endometrial MSCs that was designed for POP repair was also shown to reduce inflammatory cell infiltration and increase neovascularization in a rat model in 2013 [67].

Our own group in Sheffield has also been developing biomaterials and tissue engineered substitutes to be used in pelvic floor repair over the last 6 years. To produce the materials we have selected the technique of electrospinning. Electrospinning is a widely used technique in tissue engineering that allows fabrication of scaffolds with micro/nano sized fibers with different compositions and configurations. With respect to choice of materials for POP we have suggested a biodegradable material, poly-L-lactic acid (PLA). This is a polymer of lactic acid which is among the most commonly used polymers in biomedical applications [68]. For a biomaterial to treat stress urinary incontinence (SUI) we have selected a nondegradable polymer of polyurethane Z3-as this is not the subject of this chapter this will not be discussed further in this review.

PLA is highly biocompatible and as a degradable polymer it is commonly used as a drug delivery material [69]. In one of our first studies with a biodegradable PLA scaffold produced using the electrospinning technique we showed that the material was extensively infiltrated by host cells together with new collagen deposition and new blood vessel formation after 7 days of implantation into the rat abdomen [70]. We than tried to mimic the organization of the natural extracellular matrix by spinning transversely, obliquely and irregularly aligned PLA electrospun fibers. Here we sought to achieve the viscoelastic mechanical properties of native fascia. We confirmed that MSC cells would grow on these fibers and produce new extracellular matrix. This allowed us to report in 2016 that electrospun scaffolds with several layers of different polymers to achieve the desired biomechanical properties of native fascia [71] maintained good mechanical integrity, compared to PPL meshes, over 90 days following implantation using a rabbit model [50]. The host response to these multi-layered PLA scaffolds was characterized as a predominantly M2 (remodeling) type 30 and 90 days after implantation onto the abdomen of the rabbit.

Another crucial requirement to achieve a rapid integration into host issues is related to vascular supply in and around the biomaterial. This can be particularly concerning in cases where the wound bed is already poorly vascularized, such as pelvic floor tissues of postmenopausal women with SUI and POP [72]. The growth of new blood vessels into a tissue engineered substitute is crucial to improve its' tissue integration and to obtain a successful long term clinical outcome. It has been estimated that a distance of less than 200 μM from the supplying capillary is the critical distance for diffusion of oxygen and nutrients to any new tissue introduced into the body. Because of this, the survival of any three-dimensional tissue graft relies on rapid development of new blood vessels to supply not only the center but also the margins of the graft [73].

Accordingly we have explored the introduction of clinically acceptable agents (specifically ascorbic acid and estradiol) that would stimulate neovascularisation and new extra cellular matrix production by the patient's endogenous cells. To this end we have demonstrated effective pharmacological functionalization of electrospun PLA scaffolds by incorporating ascorbic acid into them to stimulate ECM production without compromising mechanical properties [74]. We have also recently described an estradiol releasing, biocompatible mesh of electrospun PLA which doubled the number of blood vessels in and around the mesh when tested *in vivo* [75].

8. Conclusion

Polypropylene based vaginal meshes were never designed or tested specifically for use in the pelvic floor. The complications associated with the use of these vaginal mesh implants are largely due to a poor choice of material. A basic understanding of the material properties in relation to the physiological requirements of the site of implantation is essential for those developing and evaluating materials to assist surgeons seeking to repair the weakened pelvic floor.

A major limitation here is the relative infancy of the field of urogynecology and our current inability to characterize the biomechanical features of the pelvic floor. Despite this there are now a small number of academic groups (and a very few number of commercial manufacturers) worldwide engaged in understanding the biomechanical challenges of the pelvic floor, the host response to implanted materials and how to develop biomaterials which will be designed specifically for use in the pelvic floor to be introduced on their own or with patient derived cells.

Although it is too soon for any of these approaches to have translated into clinical trials there are now alternative materials which have been rigorously evaluated *in vitro* for mechanical properties and these are starting to be evaluated in appropriate models (the sheep in Europe and monkeys in the US) which can discriminate between materials which will fail mechanically or provoke sustained inflammation and those which do not. There is now reason for optimism that better materials can and will be developed which can translate into more effective surgical support for patients without causing the unacceptably high level of severe side-effects which patients are currently suffering with PPL mesh.

Acknowledgements

We thank The Urology Foundation and the Rosetrees Trust for supporting Naside Mangir.

Author details

Naşide Mangir[1,2], Christopher R. Chapple[2] and Sheila MacNeil[1]*

*Address all correspondence to: s.macneil@sheffield.ac.uk

1 Department of Material Science and Engineering, Kroto Research Institute, University of Sheffield, UK

2 Department of Urology, Royal Hallamshire Hospital, Sheffield, UK

References

[1] Haylen BT, de Ridder D, Freeman RM, Swift SE, Berghmans B, Lee J, et al. An International Urogynecological Association (IUGA)/International Continence Society (ICS) joint report on the terminology for female pelvic floor dysfunction. International Urogynecology Journal [Internet]. Jan 25, 2010;**21**(1):5-26. Available from: http://www.ncbi.nlm.nih.gov/pubmed/19937315 [Accessed: Mar 18, 2018]

[2] Durnea CM, Khashan AS, Kenny LC, Durnea UA, Smyth MM, O'Reilly BA. Prevalence, etiology and risk factors of pelvic organ prolapse in premenopausal primiparous women. International Urogynecology Journal [Internet]. Nov 16, 2014;**25**(11):1463-1470. Available from: http://www.ncbi.nlm.nih.gov/pubmed/24737300 [Accessed: Mar 18, 2018]

[3] Smith FJ, Holman CDJ, Moorin RE, Tsokos N. Lifetime risk of undergoing surgery for pelvic organ prolapse. Obstetrics & Gynecology [Internet]. Nov 2010;**116**(5):1096-1100. Available from: http://www.ncbi.nlm.nih.gov/pubmed/20966694 [Accessed: Mar 18, 2018]

[4] Swift SE, Tate SB, Nicholas J. Correlation of symptoms with degree of pelvic organ support in a general population of women: What is pelvic organ prolapse? American Journal of Obstetrics & Gynecology [Internet]. Aug 2003;**189**(2):372-379. Available from: http://www.ncbi.nlm.nih.gov/pubmed/14520198 [Accessed: Mar 18, 2018]

[5] Wu JM, Hundley AF, Fulton RG, Myers ER. Forecasting the prevalence of pelvic floor disorders in U.S. women. Obstetrics & Gynecology [Internet]. Dec 2009;**114**(6):1278-1283. Available from: http://www.ncbi.nlm.nih.gov/pubmed/19935030 [Accessed: Mar 18, 2018]

[6] Maher C, Feiner B, Baessler K, Adams EJ, Hagen S, Glazener CM. Surgical management of pelvic organ prolapse in women. In: Maher C, editor. Cochrane Database of Systematic Reviews [Internet]. Apr 14, 2010;**4**:CD004014. DOI: http://doi.wiley.com/10.1002/14651858.CD004014.pub4 [Accessed: Feb 23, 2018]

[7] Abed H, Rahn DD, Lowenstein L, Balk EM, Clemons JL, Rogers RG, et al. Incidence and management of graft erosion, wound granulation, and dyspareunia following vaginal prolapse repair with graft materials: A systematic review. International Urogynecology Journal [Internet]. Jul 22, 2011;**22**(7):789-798. Available from: http://www.ncbi.nlm.nih.gov/pubmed/21424785 [Accessed: Feb 23, 2018]

[8] Chapple CR, Raz S, Brubaker L, Zimmern PE. Mesh sling in an era of uncertainty: lessons learned and the way forward. European Urology [Internet]. Oct 2013;**64**(4):525-529. Available from: http://www.ncbi.nlm.nih.gov/pubmed/23856039 [Accessed: Mar 2, 2018]

[9] Derbyshire V. Vaginal mesh implants: Hundreds sue NHS over "barbaric" treatment. BBC News [Internet]. Apr 18, 2017. Available from: http://www.bbccouk/news/health-39567240

[10] FDA. Food and Drug Administration. FDA safety communication: Urogynecologic surgical mesh: Update on the safety and effectiveness of transvaginal placement for pelvic organ prolapse. Review Literature and Arts of the Americas [Internet]. Jul 2011. Available from: https://www.fda.gov/downloads/MedicalDevices/Safety/AlertsandNotices/UCM262760.pdf [Accessed: Mar 12, 2018]

[11] Mahon J, Cikalo M, Varley D, Glanville J. Summaries of the Safety/Adverse Effects of Vaginal Tapes/Slings/Meshes for Stress Urinary Incontinence and Prolapse Final Report. 2012. Available from: http://www.mhra.gov.uk/home/groups/comms-ic/documents/websiteresources/con205383.pdf [Accessed: Mar 18, 2018]

[12] Epstein M, Emri I, Hartemann P, Hoet P, Leitgeb N, Martínez Martínez L, et al., Scientific Committee on Emerging and Newly Identified Health Risks. The safety of surgical meshes used in urogynecological surgery. Scientific Committee Members. Available from: http://ec.europa.eu/health/scientific_committees/emerging/Opinions/index_en.htm [Accessed: Mar 18, 2018]

[13] Food and Drug Administration, HHS. Obstetrical and Gynecological Devices; Reclassification of Surgical Mesh for Transvaginal Pelvic Organ Prolapse Repair; Final order. Federal Register [Internet]. Jan 5 2016;**81**(2):353-361. Available from: http://www.ncbi.nlm.nih.gov/pubmed/26742182 [Accessed: Mar 2, 2018]

[14] Skoczylas LC, Turner LC, Wang L, Winger DG, Shepherd JP. Changes in prolapse surgery trends relative to FDA notifications regarding vaginal mesh. International Urogynecology Journal [Internet]. Apr 1, 2014;**25**(4):471-477. Available from: http://www.ncbi.nlm.nih.gov/pubmed/24081497 [Accessed: Mar 18, 2018]

[15] Rac G, Younger A, Clemens JQ, Kobashi K, Khan A, Nitti V, et al. Stress urinary incontinence surgery trends in academic female pelvic medicine and reconstructive surgery urology practice in the setting of the food and drug administration public health notifications. Neurourology and Urodynamics [Internet]. 2017;**36**(4):1155-1160. Available from: http://www.ncbi.nlm.nih.gov/pubmed/27460448 [Accessed: Mar 18, 2018]

[16] Chapple CR, Cruz F, Deffieux X, Milani AL, Arlandis S, Artibani W, et al. Consensus Statement of the European Urology Association and the European Urogynaecological Association on the use of implanted materials for treating pelvic organ prolapse and stress urinary incontinence. European Urology [Internet]. Sep 2017;**72**(3):424-431. Available from: http://www.ncbi.nlm.nih.gov/pubmed/28413126 [Accessed: Feb 26, 2018]

[17] Brubaker L, Maher C, Jacquetin B, Rajamaheswari N, von Theobald P, Norton P. Surgery for pelvic organ prolapse. Female Pelvic Medicine & Reconstructive Surgery [Internet]. Jan 2010;**16**(1):9-19. Available from: http://www.ncbi.nlm.nih.gov/pubmed/22453085 [Accessed: Mar 18, 2018]

[18] Rutman MP, Blaivas JG. Surgery for stress urinary incontinence: Historical review. In: Continence [Internet]. London: Springer; 2009. pp. 117-132. Available from: http://link.springer.com/10.1007/978-1-84628-510-3_10 [Accessed: Mar 9, 2018]

[19] Gilbert T, Sellaro T, Badylak S. Decellularization of tissues and organs. Biomaterials [Internet]. Mar 7, 2006;**27**(19):3675-3683. Available from: http://www.ncbi.nlm.nih.gov/pubmed/16519932 [Accessed: Mar 18, 2018]

[20] Claerhout F, De Ridder D, Van Beckevoort D, Coremans G, Veldman J, Lewi P, Deprest J. Sacrocolpopexy using xenogenic acellular collagen in patients at increased risk for graft-related complications. Neurourol. Urodyn. 2010;**29**:563-567. DOI: 10.1002/nau.20805

[21] Quiroz LH, Gutman RE, Shippey S, Cundiff GW, Sanses T, Blomquist JL, et al. Abdominal sacrocolpopexy: Anatomic outcomes and complications with pelvicol, autologous and synthetic graft materials. American Journal of Obstetrics & Gynecology [Internet]. May 2008;**198**(5):557.e1-557.e5. Available from: http://linkinghub.elsevier.com/retrieve/pii/S0002937808001105 [Accessed: Mar 18, 2018]

[22] Altman D, Anzen B, Brismar S, Lopez A, Zetterström J. Long-term outcome of abdominal sacrocolpopexy using xenograft compared with synthetic mesh. Urology [Internet]. Apr 2006;**67**(4):719-724. Available from: http://www.ncbi.nlm.nih.gov/pubmed/16566983 [Accessed: Mar 18, 2018]

[23] Czerny V. Beiträge zur operativen Chirurgie. 1878. Available from: https://scholar.google.co.uk/scholar?hl=en&as_sdt=0%2C5&q=Czerny+V%3A+Beitrage+zur+Operativen+Chirurgie.+Stuttgart%3A+Verlag+von+Ferdinand+Enke%3B+1878.&btnG= [Accessed: Feb 23, 2018]

[24] Meyer IX W. The implantation of silver filigree for the closure of large hernia apertures. Annals of Surgery [Internet]. Nov 1902;**36**(5):767-778. Available from: http://www.ncbi.nlm.nih.gov/pubmed/17861212 [Accessed: Feb 25, 2018]

[25] Validire J, Imbaud P, Dutet D, Duron JJ. Large abdominal incisional hernias: repair by fascial approximation reinforced with a stainless steel mesh. British Journal of Surgery [Internet]. Jan 1986;**73**(1):8-10. Available from: http://www.ncbi.nlm.nih.gov/pubmed/2936419 [Accessed: Mar 18, 2018]

[26] Pandit AS, Henry JA. Design of surgical meshes – An engineering perspective. Technology and Health Care [Internet]. 2004;**12**(1):51-65. Available from: http://www.ncbi.nlm.nih.gov/pubmed/15096687 [Accessed: Feb 26, 2018]

[27] Usher FC. Hernia repair with knitted polypropylene mesh. Surgery, Gynecology & Obstetrics [Internet]. Aug 1963;**117**:239-240. Available from: http://www.ncbi.nlm.nih.gov/pubmed/14048019 [Accessed: Mar 18, 2018]

[28] Flum DR, Horvath K, Koepsell T. Have outcomes of incisional hernia repair improved with time? A population-based analysis. Annals of Surgery [Internet]. Jan 2003;**237**(1):129-135. Available from: http://www.ncbi.nlm.nih.gov/pubmed/12496540 [Accessed: Feb 23, 2018]

[29] Flynn WJ, Brant AE, Nelson GG. A four and one-half year analysis of tantalum gauze used in the repair of ventral hernia. Annals of Surgery [Internet]. Dec;**134**(6):1027-1034. Available from: http://www.ncbi.nlm.nih.gov/pubmed/17859504 1951[Accessed: Feb 25, 2018]

[30] Moloney GE, Gill WG, Barclay RC. Operations for hernia; technique of nylon darn. Lancet (London, England) [Internet]. Jul 10, 1948;**2**(6515):45-48. Available from: http://www.ncbi.nlm.nih.gov/pubmed/18870102 [Accessed: Feb 25, 2018]

[31] Ulmsten U, Petros P. Intravaginal slingplasty (IVS): an ambulatory surgical procedure for treatment of female urinary incontinence. Scandinavian Journal of Urology and Nephrology [Internet]. Mar 1995;**29**(1):75-82. Available from: http://www.ncbi.nlm.nih.gov/pubmed/7618052 [Accessed: Feb 25, 2018]

[32] Dällenbach P. To mesh or not to mesh: A review of pelvic organ reconstructive surgery. International Journal of Women's Health [Internet]. 2015;**7**:331-343. Available from: http://www.ncbi.nlm.nih.gov/pubmed/25848324 [Accessed: Feb 25, 2018]

[33] Usher FC, Gannon JP. Marlex mesh, a new plastic mesh for replacing tissue defects. I. Experimental studies. A.M.A. Archives of Surgery [Internet]. Jan 1959;**78**(1):131-137. Available from: http://www.ncbi.nlm.nih.gov/pubmed/13605404 [Accessed: Feb 25, 2018]

[34] Klinge U, Klosterhalfen B, Conze J, Limberg W, Obolenski B, Öttinger AP, et al. Modified mesh for hernia repair that is adapted to the physiology of the abdominal wall. European Journal of Surgery [Internet]. Nov 27, 2003;**164**(12):951-960. Available from: http://www.ncbi.nlm.nih.gov/pubmed/10029391 [Accessed: Mar 18, 2018]

[35] Klosterhalfen B, Klinge U, Schumpelick V. Functional and morphological evaluation of different polypropylene-mesh modifications for abdominal wall repair. Biomaterials [Internet]. Dec 1998;**19**(24):2235-2246. Available from: http://www.ncbi.nlm.nih.gov/pubmed/9884036 [Accessed: Mar 18, 2018]

[36] Schmidbauer S, Ladurner R, Hallfeldt KK, Mussack T. Heavy-weight versus low-weight polypropylene meshes for open sublay mesh repair of incisional hernia. European Journal of Medical Research [Internet]. Jun 22, 2005;**10**(6):247-253. Available from: http://www.ncbi.nlm.nih.gov/pubmed/16033714 [Accessed: Feb 25, 2018]

[37] Lu Y, Dong S, Chen Y, Zhang P, Tong X. Fabrication, characterization and application of polypropylene macroporous mesh for repairing pelvic floor defects. Textile Research Journal [Internet]. May 22, 2017;**87**(7):878-888. DOI: http://journals.sagepub.com/doi/10.1177/0040517516639833 [Accessed: Feb 25, 2018]

[38] Faulk DM, Londono R, Wolf MT, Ranallo CA, Carruthers CA, Wildemann JD, et al. ECM hydrogel coating mitigates the chronic inflammatory response to polypropylene mesh. Biomaterials [Internet]. Oct 2014;**35**(30):8585-8595. Available from: http://www.ncbi.nlm.nih.gov/pubmed/25043571 [Accessed: Feb 25, 2018]

[39] Read RC. Milestones in the history of hernia surgery: Prosthetic repair. Hernia [Internet]. Feb 1, 2004;**8**(1):8-14. Available from: http://www.ncbi.nlm.nih.gov/pubmed/14586774 [Accessed: Mar 18, 2018]

[40] Binnebösel M, Klink CD, Otto J, Conze J, Jansen PL, Anurov M, et al. Impact of mesh positioning on foreign body reaction and collagenous ingrowth in a rabbit model of open incisional hernia repair. Hernia [Internet]. Feb 5, 2010;**14**(1):71-77. Available from: http://www.ncbi.nlm.nih.gov/pubmed/19890675 [Accessed: Feb 23, 2018]

[41] Hayes A, Leithy M, Loulah M, Greida H, Baker F. Sublay hernioplasty versus onlay hernioplasty in incisional hernia in diabetic patients. Menoufia Medical Journal [Internet]. 2014;**27**(2):353. Available from: http://www.mmj.eg.net/text.asp?2014/27/2/353/141708 [Accessed: Mar 18, 2018]

[42] Holihan JL, Nguyen DH, Nguyen MT, Mo J, Kao LS, Liang MK. Mesh location in open ventral hernia repair: A systematic review and network meta-analysis. World Journal of Surgery [Internet]. Jan 30, 2016;**40**(1):89-99. Available from: http://www.ncbi.nlm.nih.gov/pubmed/26423675 [Accessed: Feb 23, 2018]

[43] Timmermans L, de Goede B, van Dijk SM, Kleinrensink G-J, Jeekel J, Lange JF. Meta-analysis of sublay versus onlay mesh repair in incisional hernia surgery. American Journal of Surgery [Internet]. Jun 2014;**207**(6):980-988. Available from: http://www.ncbi.nlm.nih.gov/pubmed/24315379 [Accessed: Mar 18, 2018]

[44] Petros PE, Ulmsten UI. An integral theory of female urinary incontinence. Experimental and clinical considerations. Acta Obstetricia et Gynecologica Scandinavica. Supplement [Internet]. 1990;**153**:7-31. Available from: http://www.ncbi.nlm.nih.gov/pubmed/2093278 [Accessed: Feb 23, 2018]

[45] DeLancey JOL. Anatomie aspects of vaginal eversion after hysterectomy. American Journal of Obstetrics & Gynecology [Internet]. Jun 1, 1992;**166**(6):1717-1728. Available from: https://www.sciencedirect.com/science/article/pii/000293789291562O [Accessed: Feb 23, 2018]

[46] Eilber KS, Alperin M, Khan A, Wu N, Pashos CL, Clemens JQ, et al. Outcomes of vaginal prolapse surgery among female medicare beneficiaries. Obstetrics & Gynecology [Internet]. Nov 2013;**122**(5):981-987. Available from: http://www.ncbi.nlm.nih.gov/pubmed/24104778 [Accessed: Mar 18, 2018]

[47] Pulliam SJ, Ferzandi TR, Hota LS, Elkadry EA, Rosenblatt PL. Use of synthetic mesh in pelvic reconstructive surgery: A survey of attitudes and practice patterns of urogynecologists. International Urogynecology Journal and Pelvic Floor Dysfunction [Internet]. Dec 2007;**18**(12):1405-1408. Available from: http://www.ncbi.nlm.nih.gov/pubmed/17457509 [Accessed: Mar 12, 2018]

[48] Berger RL, Li LT, Hicks SC, Davila JA, Kao LS, Liang MK. Development and validation of a risk-stratification score for surgical site occurrence and surgical site infection after open ventral hernia repair. Journal of the American College of Surgeons [Internet]. Dec 2013;**217**(6):974-982. Available from: http://www.ncbi.nlm.nih.gov/pubmed/24051068 [Accessed: Feb 23, 2018]

[49] Manodoro S, Endo M, Uvin P, Albersen M, Vláčil J, Engels A, et al. Graft-related complications and biaxial tensiometry following experimental vaginal implantation of flat mesh of variable dimensions. BJOG: An International Journal of Obstetrics & Gynaecology [Internet]. Jan 1, 2013;**120**(2):244-250. DOI: http://doi.wiley.com/10.1111/1471-0528.12081 [Accessed: Feb 25, 2018]

[50] Roman S, Urbánková I, Callewaert G, Lesage F, Hillary C, Osman NI, et al. Evaluating alternative materials for the treatment of stress urinary incontinence and pelvic organ prolapse: A comparison of the in vivo response to meshes implanted in rabbits. Journal of Urology [Internet]. Jul 2016;**196**(1):261-269. Available from: http://www.ncbi.nlm.nih.gov/pubmed/26880411 [Accessed: Feb 25, 2018]

[51] Nolfi AL, Brown BN, Liang R, Palcsey SL, Bonidie MJ, Abramowitch SD, et al. Host response to synthetic mesh in women with mesh complications. American Journal of Obstetrics & Gynecology [Internet]. 2016;**215**(2):206.e1-206.e8. Available from: http://www.ncbi.nlm.nih.gov/pubmed/27094962 [Accessed: Mar 18, 2018]

[52] Moalli PA, Howden NS, Lowder JL, Navarro J, Debes KM, Abramowitch SD, et al. A rat model to study the structural properties of the vagina and its supportive tissues. American Journal of Obstetrics & Gynecology [Internet]. Jan 2005;**192**(1):80-88. Available from: http://www.ncbi.nlm.nih.gov/pubmed/15672007 [Accessed: Mar 18, 2018]

[53] Choe JM, Kothandapani R, James L, Bowling D. Autologous, cadaveric, and synthetic materials used in sling surgery: Comparative biomechanical analysis. Urology [Internet]. Sep 2001;**58**(3):482-486. Available from: http://www.ncbi.nlm.nih.gov/pubmed/11549510 [Accessed: Mar 18, 2018]

[54] Kruger JA, Yan X, Li X, Nielsen PM, Nash MP. Applications of Pelvic Floor Modeling and Simulation. In: Biomechanics of the Female Pelvic Floor; 2016. pp. 367-382. DOI: 10.1016/B978-0-12-803228-2.00018-0

[55] Rocha P, Parente M, Mascarenhas T, Fernandes A, Jorge RN. Effect of surgical mesh implant in the uterine prolapse correction. In: Bioengineering (ENBENG), 2015 IEEE 4th Portuguese Meeting on IEEE. Feb 26, 2015. pp. 1-4

[56] Iakovlev VV, Guelcher SA, Bendavid R. Degradation of polypropylene *in vivo*: A microscopic analysis of meshes explanted from patients. Journal of Biomedical Materials Research Part B: Applied Biomaterials [Internet]. Feb 1, 2017;**105**(2):237-248. DOI: http://doi.wiley.com/10.1002/jbm.b.33502 [Accessed: Feb 25, 2018]

[57] Talley AD, Rogers BR, Iakovlev V, Dunn RF, Guelcher SA. Oxidation and degradation of polypropylene transvaginal mesh. Journal of Biomaterials Science, Polymer Edition [Internet]. Mar 24, 2017;**28**(5):444-458. DOI: https://www.tandfonline.com/doi/full/10.1080/09205063.2017.1279045 [Accessed: Feb 25, 2018]

[58] Miklos JR, Chinthakanan O, Moore RD, Mitchell GK, Favors S, Karp DR, et al. The IUGA/ICS classification of synthetic mesh complications in female pelvic floor reconstructive surgery: a multicenter study. International Urogynecology Journal [Internet]. Jun 21, 2016;**27**(6):933-938. Available from: http://www.ncbi.nlm.nih.gov/pubmed/26690360 [Accessed: Mar 18, 2018]

[59] Giannitsas K, Costantini E. How to deal with pain following a vaginal mesh Insertion. European Urology Focus [Internet]. Aug 2016;**2**(3):268-271. Available from: http://www.ncbi.nlm.nih.gov/pubmed/28723372 [Accessed: Mar 18, 2018]

[60] Sussman EM, Halpin MC, Muster J, Moon RT, Ratner BD. Porous implants modulate healing and induce shifts in local macrophage polarization in the foreign body reaction. Annals of Biomedical Engineering [Internet]. Jul 19, 2014;**42**(7):1508-1516. Available from: http://www.ncbi.nlm.nih.gov/pubmed/24248559 [Accessed: Mar 18, 2018]

[61] Fukano Y, Usui ML, Underwood RA, Isenhath S, Marshall AJ, Hauch KD, et al. Epidermal and dermal integration into sphere-templated porous poly(2-hydroxyethyl methacrylate) implants in mice. Journal of Biomedical Materials Research Part A [Internet]. Sep 15, 2010;**9999A**(4)s. Available from: http://www.ncbi.nlm.nih.gov/pubmed/20694984 [Accessed: Mar 18, 2018]

[62] Feola A, Abramowitch S, Jallah Z, Stein S, Barone W, Palcsey S, et al. Deterioration in biomechanical properties of the vagina following implantation of a high-stiffness prolapse mesh. BJOG: An International Journal of Obstetrics & Gynaecology [Internet]. Jan 2013;**120**(2):224-232. Available from: http://www.ncbi.nlm.nih.gov/pubmed/23240801 [Accessed: Mar 18, 2018]

[63] Todros S, Pavan PG, Natali AN. Biomechanical properties of synthetic surgical meshes for pelvic prolapse repair. Journal of the Mechanical Behavior of Biomedical Materials [Internet]. Mar 2016;**55**:271-285. Available from: http://www.ncbi.nlm.nih.gov/pubmed/26615384 [Accessed: Mar 18, 2018]

[64] Hung M-J, Wen M-C, Hung C-N, Ho ES-C, Chen G-D, Yang VC. Tissue-engineered fascia from vaginal fibroblasts for patientsneeding reconstructive pelvic surgery. International Urogynecology Journal [Internet]. Sep 18, 2010;**21**(9):1085-1093. Available from: http://www.ncbi.nlm.nih.gov/pubmed/20480140 [Accessed: Mar 18, 2018]

[65] Li Q, Wang J, Liu H, Xie B, Wei L. Tissue-engineered mesh for pelvic floor reconstruction fabricated from silk fibroin scaffold with adipose-derived mesenchymal stem ells. Cell and Tissue Research [Internet]. Nov 2013;**354**(2):471-480. Available from: http://www.ncbi.nlm.nih.gov/pubmed/23996203 [Accessed: Mar 18, 2018]

[66] Ulrich D, Edwards SL, White JF, Supit T, Ramshaw JAM, Lo C, et al. A preclinical evaluation of alternative synthetic biomaterials for fascial defect repair using a rat abdominal hernia model. In: Neves NM, editor. PLoS One [Internet]. Nov 20, 2012;**7**(11):e50044. Available from: http://www.ncbi.nlm.nih.gov/pubmed/23185528 [Accessed: Feb 25, 2018]

[67] Ulrich D, Edwards SL, Su K, Tan KS, White JF, Ramshaw JAM, et al. Human endometrial mesenchymal stem cells modulate the tissue response and mechanical behavior of polyamide mesh implants for pelvic organ prolapse repair. Tissue Engineering Part A [Internet]. Feb 2014;**20**(3-4):785-798. Available from: http://www.ncbi.nlm.nih.gov/pubmed/24083684 [Accessed: Feb 25, 2018]

[68] Lasprilla AJR, Martinez GAR, Lunelli BH, Jardini AL, Filho RM. Poly-lactic acid synthesis for application in biomedical devices — A review. Biotechnology Advances [Internet]. Jan 2012;**30**(1):321-328. Available from: http://www.ncbi.nlm.nih.gov/pubmed/21756992 [Accessed: Feb 25, 2018]

[69] Fredenberg S, Wahlgren M, Reslow M, Axelsson A. The mechanisms of drug release in poly(lactic-co-glycolic acid)-based drug delivery systems—A review. International Journal of Pharmaceutics [Internet]. Aug 30, 2011;**415**(1-2):34-52. Available from: http://www.ncbi.nlm.nih.gov/pubmed/21640806 [Accessed: Feb 25, 2018]

[70] Roman Regueros S, Albersen M, Manodoro S, Zia S, Osman NI, Bullock AJ, et al. Acute *in vivo* response to an alternative implant for urogynecology. BioMed Research International [Internet]. 2014;**2014**:1-10. Available from: http://www.ncbi.nlm.nih.gov/pubmed/25136633 [Accessed: Feb 25, 2018]

[71] Roman S, Mangir N, Bissoli J, Chapple CR, MacNeil S. Biodegradable scaffolds designed to mimic fascia-like properties for the treatment of pelvic organ prolapse and stress urinary incontinence. Journal of Biomaterials Applications [Internet]. May 18, 2016;**30**(10):1578-1588. DOI: http://journals.sagepub.com/doi/10.1177/0885328216633373 [Accessed: Feb 23, 2018]

[72] Semmens JP, Wagner G. Estrogen deprivation and vaginal function in postmenopausal women. Journal of the American Medical Association [Internet]. Jul 23, 1982;**248**(4):445-448. Available from: http://www.ncbi.nlm.nih.gov/pubmed/6283189 [Accessed: Feb 25, 2018]

[73] Rouwkema J, Rivron NC, van Blitterswijk CA. Vascularization in tissue engineering. Trends in Biotechnology [Internet]. Aug 2008;**26**(8):434-441. Available from: http://www.ncbi.nlm.nih.gov/pubmed/18585808 [Accessed: Mar 18, 2018]

[74] Mangır N, Bullock AJ, Roman S, Osman N, Chapple C, MacNeil S. Production of ascorbic acid releasing biomaterials for pelvic floor repair. Acta Biomaterialia [Internet]. Jan 2016;**29**:188-197. Available from: http://www.ncbi.nlm.nih.gov/pubmed/26478470 [Accessed: Feb 25, 2018]

[75] Mangır N, Hillary CJ, Chapple CR, MacNeil S. Oestradiol-releasing Biodegradable Mesh Stimulates Collagen Production and Angiogenesis: An Approach to Improving Biomaterial Integration in Pelvic Floor Repair. European urology focus. 2017 Jun 3: pii: S2405-4569(17)30122-0. DOI: 10.1016/j.euf.2017.05.004

Chapter 5

Recurrent Pelvic Organ Prolapse

Nidhi Sharma and Sudakshina Chakrabarti

Additional information is available at the end of the chapter

http://dx.doi.org/10.5772/intechopen.76669

Abstract

The treatment of recurrent pelvic organ prolapse is challenging. The pelvic floor symptom needs to be treated, a high quality of life has to be ensured and complications have to be minimized. There is a wide range of surgical options that may be used. The surgeon should be able to discuss and offer native tissue procedures for prolapse. In addition, for the clinically challenging situations of recurrent prolapse, mesh augmented procedures may need to be discussed with the patient. A thorough knowledge of mesh and graft options, as well as knowledge of prolapse recurrence and adverse events rate, can help guide clinicians in counseling their patients effectively. Ultimately, this will allow surgeons to choose a personalized treatment option that best align with a woman's lifestyle and treatment goals. In this chapter the anatomical concepts of supports of vagina are elaborated. The pelvic diaphragm, lateral attachment of vagina to arcus tendineus fascia pelvis, intrinsic and extrinsic sphincter control mechanisms are elaborated. The surgical techniques of suspending the vaginal vault with autologous tissue and synthetic mesh are discussed. Finally, the role of minimally invasive surgery of pelvic floor is discussed as an integral part of management of recurrent vaginal prolapse.

Keywords: recurrent POP, pelvic floor, perineum, prolapse, vaginal vault prolapse, sacrospinous fixation

1. Introduction

Vaginal prolapse can be studied in defects at three levels of Prof John Delancey (**Figure 1**).

Usually vault prolapse is associated with anterior and/or posterior wall prolapse. The anterior compartment, the central compartment and the posterior compartment defect. Anterior compartment consists of the bladder and urethra. The central compartment consists of the vaginal vault/uterus. The rectum and perineal body form the posterior compartment. The lateral

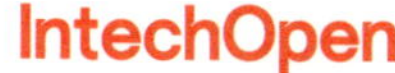

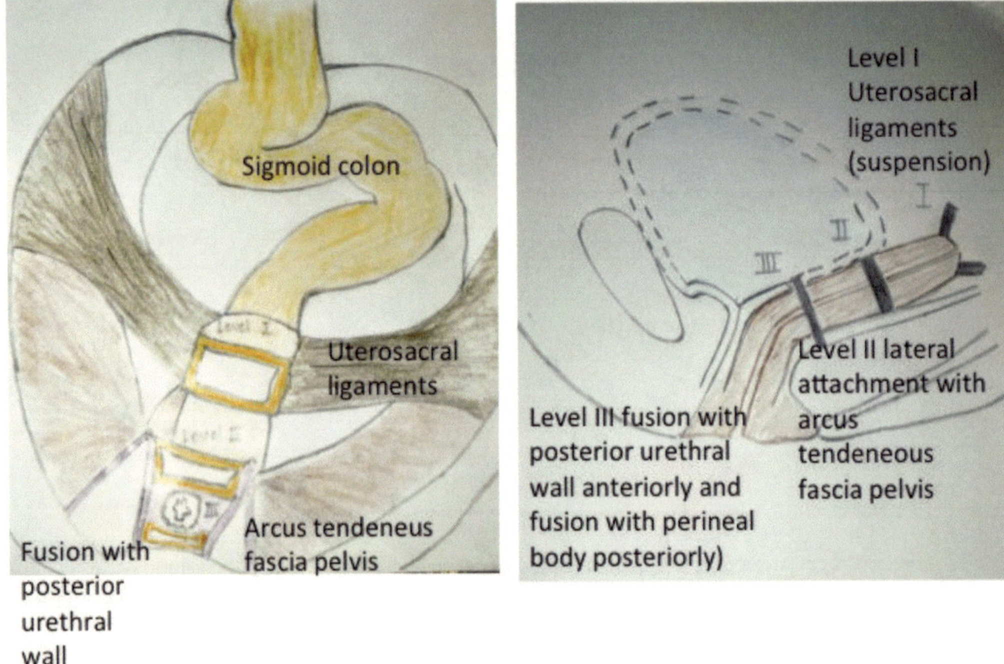

Figure 1. Professor John De Lancey's support of vaginal vault after hysterectomy as viewed from above and laterally.

compartment defect is the detachment from the arcus tendineus fascia pelvis. The enterocele and posterior compartment dysfunction is the commonest form of post hysterectomy vaginal vault prolapse (**Figure 2**).

Vault prolapse can occur following hysterectomy done for non-prolapse indications if the surgeon at the time of vaginal vault closure does not perform the vault suspension procedure. At the time of abdominal hysterectomy done for benign gynecological diseases like fibroid, adenomyosis, dysfunctional uterine bleeding, the uterosacral ligaments are clamped cut and ligated. The vaginal vault is sutured. This sutured vaginal vault needs to be suspended to the stumps of uterosacral ligaments to support the vagina following hysterectomy. This vital step is the most important point to be remembered by general gynecology practitioners to prevent the occurrence of vault prolapse following hysterectomy.

Recurrent pelvic organ prolapse can be defined as

"The recurrent complaint of something coming down pervaginum, following hysterectomy done for pelvic organ prolapse or other benign gynecological indications". Unfortunately this definition does not take into account the wide variation in this symptom and the underlying etiology. Some women may be asymptomatic while others may have severe symptoms.

Severity and quantity of symptoms that should be considered in history are:

1. Duration of complaint and whether the problem has been worsening

2. Presence of triggering factors or events (e.g. Coughing, sneezing, lifting, bending, feeling of urgency)

3. Constant or intermittent urine loss and provocation by minimal increase in intraabdominal pressure. Such as movement, changes in position, and incontinence with an empty bladder

4. Associated frequency, urgency, dysuria, pain with a full bladder, and a history of urinary tract infections

5. Concomitant symptoms of fecal incontinence or rectal prolapse

6. Indication of previous Hysterectomy and coexisting complicating or exacerbating medical problems like diabetes

7. Obstetrical history, including difficult deliveries, episiotomy, grand multiparty, forceps use, obstetrical lacerations, and large babies

8. Type of previous pelvic surgeries, especially the incontinence procedures, hysterectomy, or pelvic floor reconstructive procedures

9. History of spinal and central nervous system surgeries

10. Lifestyle issues like smoking, alcohol or caffeine abuse, and occupational and recreational factors causing severe or repetitive increase in intraabdominal pressure

11. Patients with coexisting pelvic organ prolapse may report dyspareunia, vaginal pain on ambulation, and a bulging sensation in vagina

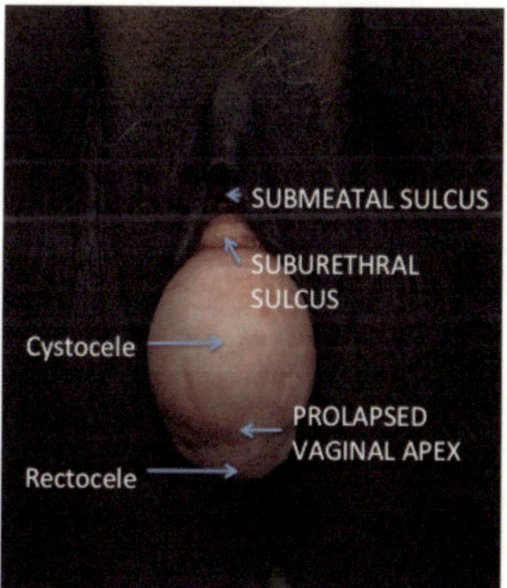

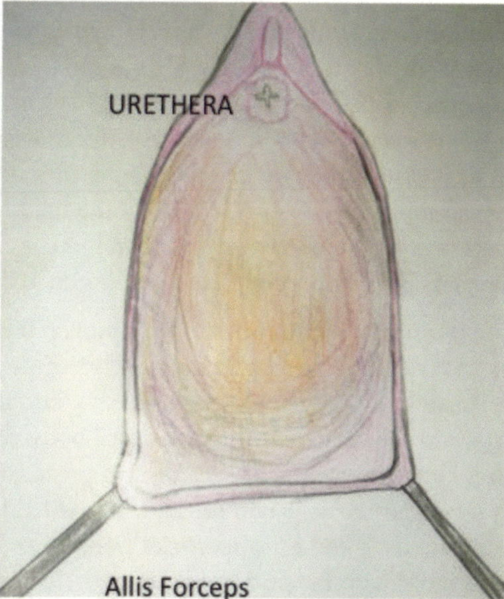

Figure 2. Vaginal vault prolapse with cystocele and enterocele (Submeatal sulcus and suburethral sulcus is maintained). The leading point of the prolapse is the prolapsed vaginal apex hence also called as apical vaginal prolapse. Diagrammatic representation of the vaginal vault prolapse: the edges of the vaginal apex are held by Allis tissue holding forceps.

2. Anatomical considerations

In 1555 Andreas Vesalius referred to the pelvic floor muscles as "Musculus sedem attollens". Von Behr later referred this as levator ani. The term pelvic diaphragm includes ischiococcygeus, ileococcygeus and pubococcygeus which all forms the levator ani. Puborectalis or "Sphincter Recti" is described as the fibers of pubococcygeus which loop around the rectum and this muscle is now included in the levator ani group. As the muscles of the pelvic diaphragm are intimately related to the urethra, vagina, rectum and anal canal, the term pubovisceralis for the muscles of pelvic floor was first coined by Lawson and was later supported by Delancey [1–3].

The muscles in pelvis can be classified into two groups. The lateral wall muscles and the pelvic floor muscles. The lateral wall muscles include the obturator internus and piriformis and the pelvic floor muscles include the levator ani. The pelvic floor muscles form the pelvic diaphragm [4, 5]. The levator ani is a broad thin sheet of muscle arising from the inner aspect of the pelvic walls unites with its fellow from the opposite side to form the floor of pelvic cavity. It supports the pelvic viscera and some of its fibers get attached to the wall of the visceral structures passing through it. The levator ani has an extensive origin starting from the posterior surface of the superior ramus of pubic bone, obturator fascia to the inner aspect of the ischial spine. The fibers pass downward and backwards thus creating a shallow saucer like structure on which the pelvic viscera rests. The posterior most fibers from either side get attached to the sides of the terminal two pieces of coccyx. Fibers immediately anterior to this unite with the fellow fibers of opposite side to form a median anococcygeal raphe extending between the coccyx and the posterior margin of anus.

The term pubovisceralis is extensively used in gynecological texts but it is not commonly mentioned in anatomical texts. The portions of pubovisceralis that are inserted into the urethra, vagina, perineal body and anal canal were given names as pubourethralis, pubovaginalis and puboperinalis respectively by Lawson [4–6]. The action of these muscles is to provide support to the visceral organs. The ileococcygeous muscle provides support to the posterior compartment and fuses anterior to the coccyx with fibers of opposite side to form the anococcygeal raphe or the levator plate in the median plane. This thin muscular plate supports the viscera of the pelvis especially when there is rise in intraabdominal pressure. Sagging of levator plate is an important defect leading to loss of support of the pelvic organs [7, 8].

The perineal body, which lies posterior to the posterior vaginal wall and anterior to the wall of anal canal, is an important support of pelvic floor. The attachments and components of perineal body are still debated. Recent studies using 3D endovaginal ultrasonography have assessed the structure of the perineal body showed that it has mixed echogenicity and situated between rectum, anal canal and posterior wall of vagina [2, 5]. Perineal body is divided into two levels, i.e. a superficial level which is continuous with external anal sphincter, bulbospongiosus and the superficial transverse perineal muscles and a deeper part, which is in continuity with the pubovisceralis muscle of the pelvic floor [6, 7].

The endopelvic connective tissue in this area attaches to the perineal membrane and laterally it stretches over the levator ani and condenses to form the arcus tendineus fascia pelvis, which stretches from pubic bone till the ischial spine. This arcus tendineus fascia pelvis lies at the junction of the fascia of the obturator internus and levator ani muscle. This tissue provides support to vagina vault laterally [2, 8, 9].

3. Initial evaluation

The initial evaluation of patients with vaginal vault prolapse requires a systematic approach to consider the probable causes.

3.1. History

Physicians treating the recurrent prolapse patient should empathically ask them how the prolapse specially affects their life and to what degree the prolapse bothers them.

3.2. Physical examination

The physical examination of the patient with recurrent prolapse should focus on both the general medical conditions that may affect the pelvic organs as well as the problems related to prolapse [10, 11]. Such conditions include cardiovascular insufficiency, pulmonary disease, occult neurologic processes, (e.g. Multiple sclerosis, stroke, Parkinson's disease, and anomalies of the spine and lower back), abdominal masses and general activity of the patient [12, 13].

3.3. Pelvic examination

This should be performed by POP-Q system [12–14]. A special note should be made regarding pelvic organ prolapse and atrophy. Levator ani muscle symmetry should be noted during the ability to squeeze test. Anal sphincter function, presence of fissures and symmetry during squeezing should also be noted.

Recurrent prolapse assessment should include urodynamic studies to reach a correct diagnosis of the type of incontinence associated with recurrent prolapse. The indications of urodynamic studies are:

1. The diagnosis is uncertain (major discrepancies between the history, voiding diary and symptom scale).
2. Elevated post void residual urine volume.
3. Associated neurological conditions like multiple sclerosis leading to recurrent prolapse.
4. Previous surgery for incontinence correction.
5. Coexisting rectal prolapse.

3.4. Systemic examination

Gait assessment should be done and mobility status should be noted. A detailed neurological examination should incorporate measures of mental status, perineal sensation, perineal reflexes and patellar reflexes. Cardiovascular examination should be done to rule out lower extremities edema and feature of congestive heart failure [15–17].

3.5. Simple primary care tests

Simple primary care clinical tests are an integral part of initial evaluation. Pelvic Floor Distress Inventory-Short Form 20 (PFDI-20), the Pelvic Floor Impact Questionnaire-7 (PFIQ-7) and the ICIQ-VS score can be used to evaluate the quality of life and severity of symptoms. The most common questionnaire used is the PFDI-20 questionnaire [18–20].

4. Management options

The management options of recurrent pelvic organ prolapse is almost always surgical. It is to be realized that surgical options are the first choice as they provide a long-term relief. Surgical measures should always be accompanied by pelvic muscle strengthening exercises in the postoperative period for best outcome.

The surgical procedure must be case based. If the initial repair was vaginal hysterectomy with pelvic floor repair the subsequent repair can be sacrospinous colpopexy or sacrospinous fixation. If the initial repair was sacrohysteropexy the recurrent prolapse can be managed by vaginal hysterectomy, anterior colporrhaphy and posterior colpoperineorrhaphy along with McCall's culdoplasty.

Corrective Surgeries for vaginal Vault Prolapse	
Vaginal Approach	
McCall's Culdoplasty	Approximation of uterosacral ligaments and attachment of vaginal vault to uterosacral ligaments
Sacrospinous Colpopexy	Vaginal Vault to sacrospinous ligament
Ileococcygeus colpopexy	Vaginal Vault to ileococcygeous muscle
Uterosacral ligament Suspension	Vaginal Vault to uterosacral ligaments
Abdominal Approach	
Abdominal Sacrocolpopexy	Vaginal Vault to presacral periosteum
Abdominal uterosacral suspension	Vaginal Vault to uterosacral ligaments
Laparoscopic Approach	
Laparoscopic Sacrocolpopexy	Vaginal vault to presacral periosteum
Robotic Approach	
Robotic Sacrocolpopexy	Vaginal vault to presacral periosteum

Table 1. Corrective surgery for vaginal vault prolapse.

The reconstructive surgical procedures for the anterior and posterior vaginal vault prolapse are listed in **Table 1**. The anterior vaginal Wall repairs include anterior colporrhaphy and site-specific repair. The posterior vaginal wall repair procedures include posterior colporrhaphy, site-specific repair, perineorrhaphy, McCall's culdoplasty and Moskowitz procedure. The procedures for vault prolapse following hysterectomy include sacrospinous colpopexy, uterosacral ligament (USLS) suspension via abdominal or vaginal route, ileococcygeal fascia suspension and abdominal sacrocolpopexy [21].

5. Sacrospinous colpopexy

Access to sacrospinous ligament is obtained through the Para rectal space in posterior approach and through the paravesical space in the anterior approach. The right ischial spine is localized digitally and after retractor positioning the ligament is made visible through blunt dissection. Two permanent sutures (Prolene 1.0, Ethicon, Somerville, NJ, USA) are placed through the right sacrospinous ligament at least 2 cm from the ischial spine. Pulley sutures are used to anchor the undersurface of the anterior vaginal cuff (anterior sacrospinous suspension) or posterior cuff (posterior sacrospinous suspension) along the sacrospinous ligament medially and laterally. During both techniques, the medial and lateral fixation sutures are placed at least 2 cm apart along the ligament. Hereafter an additional anterior and/or posterior colporrhaphy or incontinence surgery can be performed. The procedure is acceptable with few complications [22]. Sacrospinous Fixation can be done using Miya hook or Capio (**Figure 3**).

There are two ways to access the sacrospinous ligament: the anterior approach and the posterior approach. In the anterior approach the sacrospinous ligament is accessed after dissecting the paravaginal and paravesical spaces and the anterior vaginal cuff is anchored to the sacrospinous ligament. In the posterior approach the pararectal fossa is opened after dissected the posterior vaginal wall from the rectovaginal fascia. And the posterior cuff of vagina is anchored to the sacrospinous ligament.

In the posterior approach the vaginal mucosa is incised transversely at the posterior fourchette and the posterior vaginal mucosal flap is raised above from rectovaginal fascia. The assistant deflects the rectum medially while the surgeon palpates the ischial spine and identifies the sacrospinous ligament. A Miya hook passed through the sacrospinous ligament. The Miya hook is threaded with the suture and the sutures are carried and anchored to the vaginal vault. The permanent sutures are placed through the posterior side of the vagina in the posterior approach. The lower two thirds of posterior vaginal wall is closed with absorbable sutures (Vicryl 2, Eticon Somerville, NJ, USA). The permanent sutures are now tightened and the remaining one third of the vaginal wall is also closed (**Figures 3(a)–(c)**). The same principal is applied for sacrospinous hysteropexy in an intact uterus. The posterior sacrospinous approach is less invasive but the vaginal axis is slightly downwards as compared to the physiological axis of vagina. This predisposes to anterior compartment defects as the raised intraabdominal pressures are now directly transmitted to the anterior vaginal wall.

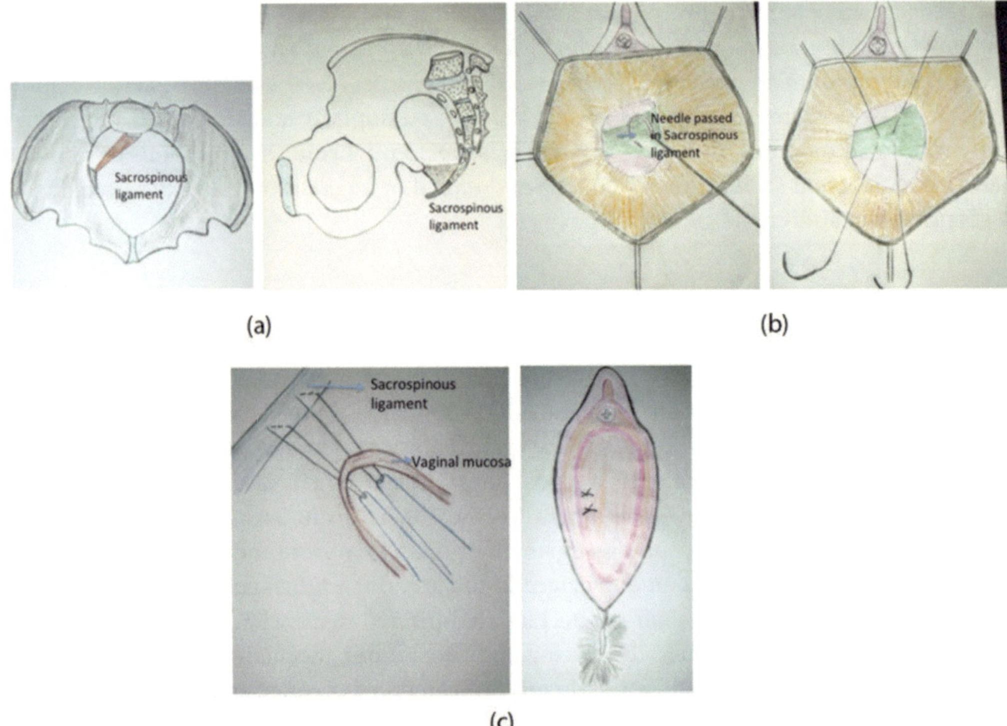

Figure 3. (a) The anatomical identification of sacrospinous ligaments as viewed from above and laterally. (b) The vaginal vault is anchored to the sacrospinous ligaments with delayed absorbable or nonabsorbable sutures. (c) The vaginal mucosa is anchored and closed.

The anterior approach was developed subsequently to overcome the shortcomings of posterior approach. In the anterior approach a vertical anterior vaginal incision is made for retro pubic entry and paravaginal and paravesical space is dissected. The sacrospinous ligament is identified and the anterior cuff of vagina is anchored with two polytetrafluoroethylene (00) sutures. The two sutures are placed 2 cm apart on sacrospinous ligament. The same procedure is performed on the contralateral sacrospinous ligament.

The anterior suspension technique positions the vaginal vault in a more capacious anatomic space, in comparison to the relatively narrow pararectal area occupied by the upper vagina after posterior sacrospinous vault suspension (**Figure 4(a)** and **(b)**). After anterior sacrospinous vaginal vault suspension, vaginal length and apical suspension are slightly increased. The axis of the suspended vagina appears more physiological. There are less chances of recurrent anterior compartment prolapse as compared with the posterior sacrospinous vaginal vault suspension procedure. The upper vaginal lumen caliber and sexual function are adequately preserved in both techniques [23]. The posterior vaginal wall laxity, on the contrary, is more common after anterior sacrospinous vault suspension.

However, these differences are likely to be influenced by differences in levator muscle tone and degree of perineal support. So a posterior colporrhaphy may be concurrently performed

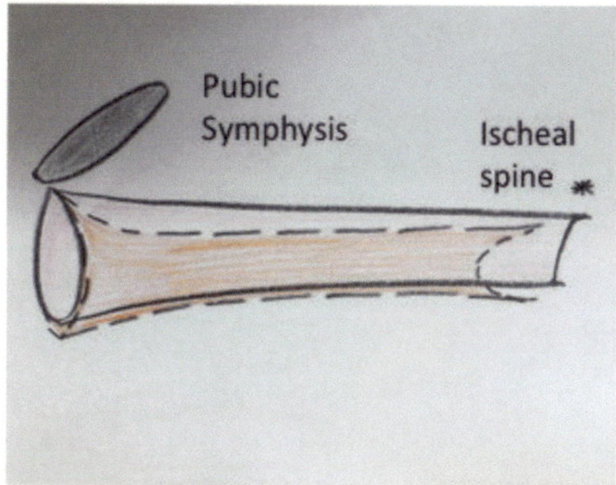

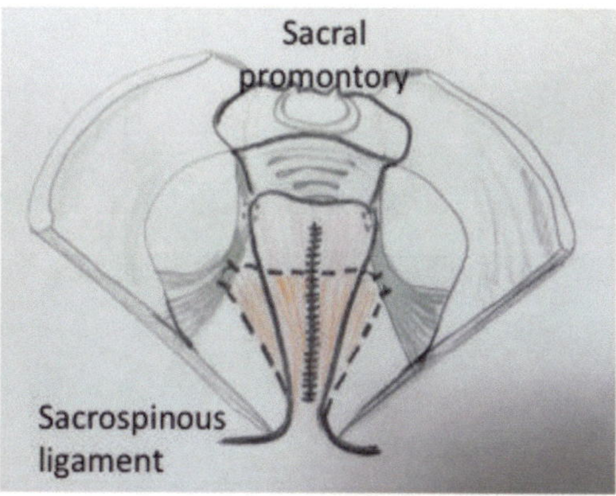

Figure 4. Anterior v/s posterior sacrospinous vault fixation: Postoperative comparison based on pelvic organ prolapse . Solid line: Anterior sacrospinous vault fixation, dashed line: Posterior sacrospinous fixation. (a): Lateral view of Vaginal axis after anterior and posterior bilateral sacrospinous fixation. (b): Anterior posterior view of vaginal axis after anterior and posterior bilateral sacrospinous fixation.

with anterior sacrospinous fixation to achieve the best outcome. Postoperative strengthening of perineal muscles by structured pelvic exercises is effective.

6. Uterosacral vaginal vault suspension

In vault prolapse the endopelvic fascia surrounding the vagina is broken at specific points. A site-specific repair and anchoring to the stumps of uterosacral ligaments will restore the suspension. Three principles are identification of the fascia defect, reducing the enterocele sac and closure of the fascia defect. Finally the vagina is anchored to the Level 1 support of uterosacral ligament making the procedure most anatomically close to physiologically correct vaginal axis.

Vaginal apex is grabbed with two Allis clamps. The vaginal mucosa over the enterocele is incised. The enterocele sac is identified and dissected till the base or neck of the sac. The enterocele sac is opened carefully and contents are reduced taking care of adhesions. The excessive peritoneum is excised. A Deaver retractor is placed anteriorly and used to pack the abdominal contents anteriorly.

The uterosacral ligament stumps are identified; remnants are usually believed to be present at 5 0′clock and 7 0′clock position. The ureter position is confirmed by palpating the pelvic sidewall. The ureter is usually placed 2–3 cm lateral and ventral to the ischial spine. A non-absorbable Prolene 1/0 suture is placed on the uterosacral remnant on left side passing the needle from lateral to medial side to avoid injuring the ureter. The rectum is then deflected away by the non-dominant hand. A second suture is placed further high and medially on the left uterosacral ligament for better anchoring. The peritoneum is included in the stich and now the stich is passed in the opposite uterosacral ligament taking the needle from lateral to medial side. Now these sutures are tied and this obliterates the cul-de-sac (**Figure 5**). Anterior colporrhaphy or sling procedures if required are performed at this stage now.

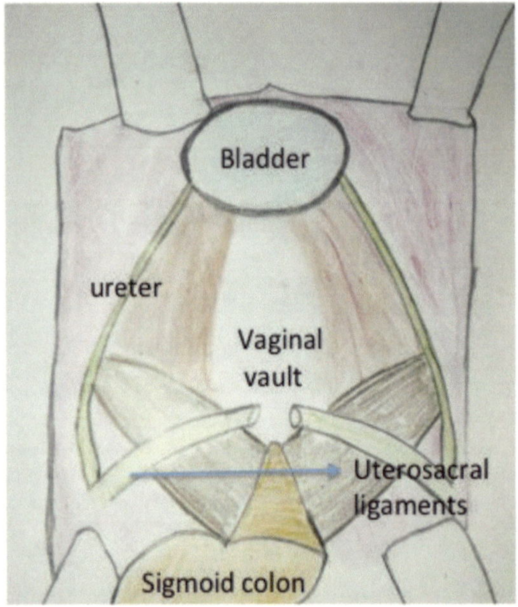

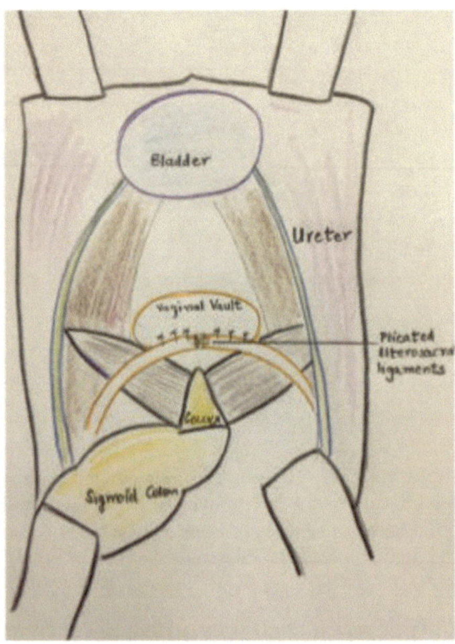

Figure 5. The abdominal uterosacral ligament suspension.

The nonabsorbable suture ends from the uterosacral ligaments are now attached to the vaginal apex. One suture end is taken through the lateral aspect of the posterior vaginal wall and the other is attached to the lateral aspect of the anterior vaginal wall. The same is repeated on the other side.

Tying these sutures suspends the vagina in the hollow of the sacrum and restores the continuity of the endopelvic fascia of the anterior and posterior vaginal walls [24].

The single most careful point in this procedure is prevention of ureteric injury or kinking. It is important to perform an intraoperative cystoscopy to ensure ureteral patency. If the urine spurt is not seen in cystoscopy then the suspension sutures on that side should be removed and ureters reevaluated. Often the anchoring can be achieved by taking a more medial suture through the uterosacral ligament.

7. Ileococcygeous fascia suspension

In 1963, Inmon used ileococcygeal fascia in three women for bilateral fixation of vaginal vault in patients with inadequate uterosacral ligaments. In 1993, Schull and colleagues had performed this technique in 42 women. The principle is to identify all fascial defects prior to surgery. Posterior perineal incision is made. The vaginal epithelium is then freed from the rectum and rectovaginalis fascia. The dissection is carried further laterally to the levators and cephalad to the vaginal cuff. The ileococcygeal muscle is identified lateral to the rectum and anterior to the ischial spine. The non-dominant hand is used to depress the rectum away from the ischial spine.

http://dx.doi.org/10.5772/intechopen.76669

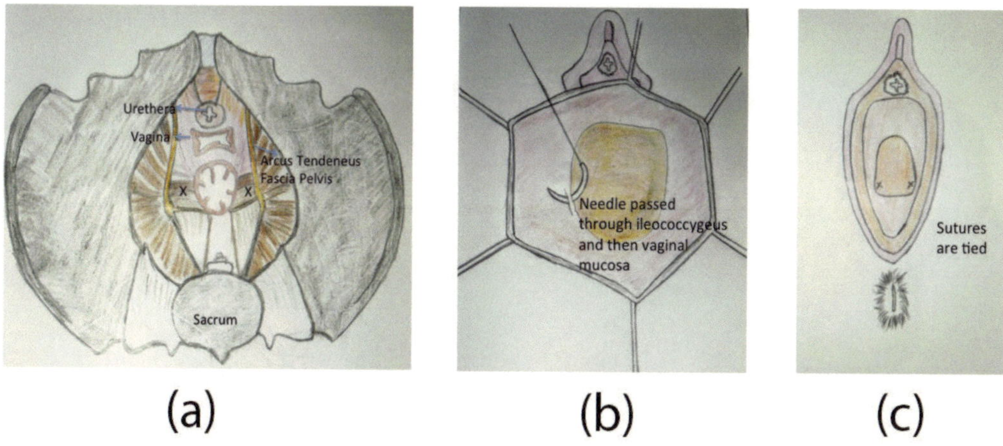

Figure 6. (a) The ileococcygeus muscle anatomical identification. (b) The ileococcygeus fixation of vaginal mucosa and closure of vagina after bilateral ileococcygeus fixation.

A suture is placed just anterior to the ischial spine in the fascia covering the ileococcygeous muscle. Both ends of the loop are now passed through the ipsilateral vaginal apex. A similar suture is placed on the contralateral ileococcygeus muscle and vaginal apex is sutured to the opposite ileococcygeus (**Figure 6(a)-(c)**). A delayed absorbable suture like Vicryl 1,0, Ethicon, Somerville, NJ, USA should pass through the entire vaginal thickness.

A specific complication is anterior vaginal wall relaxation due to non-physiological axis of the reconstructed vaginal support, which makes the vagina tilt anteriorly [25].

8. Abdominal sacrocolpopexy

Post Hysterectomy Vaginal Vault Prolapse always requires a surgical correction. The suspension of vagina in the hollow of sacrum to the anterior longitudinal ligament of first sacral vertebra has been shown to be an effective treatment of vault prolapse.

Peritoneum over vaginal apex is opened to identify the endopelvic fascia. A continuous covering of endopelvic fascia is created around the vaginal epithelium. Nonabsorbable sutures are used to suspend the vagina along with endopelvic fascia to the sacral periosteum [26].

Sacrocolpopexy is an abdominal operation that connects the top of the vagina with a strip of permanent synthetic mesh to the sacrum bone. This operation is sturdy, with many studies showing success rates of over 90%. Cutting and tying the mesh design an "inverted Y" shaped mesh.

The patient is placed in low lithotomy position to allow vaginal manipulation during the surgery. The vagina is packed with a sponge stick or an E sizer, End-to-end anastomosis **sizer** (Auto Suture EEA reusable **sizer**; United States Surgical, Tyco Healthcare Group LP, Norwalk, CT, USA).

The lower limbs of inverted Y are anchored to the full thickness of vagina by multiple interrupted sutures. The mesh is placed around half way down the anterior wall, thereby correcting the undiagnosed, unidentified cystocele.

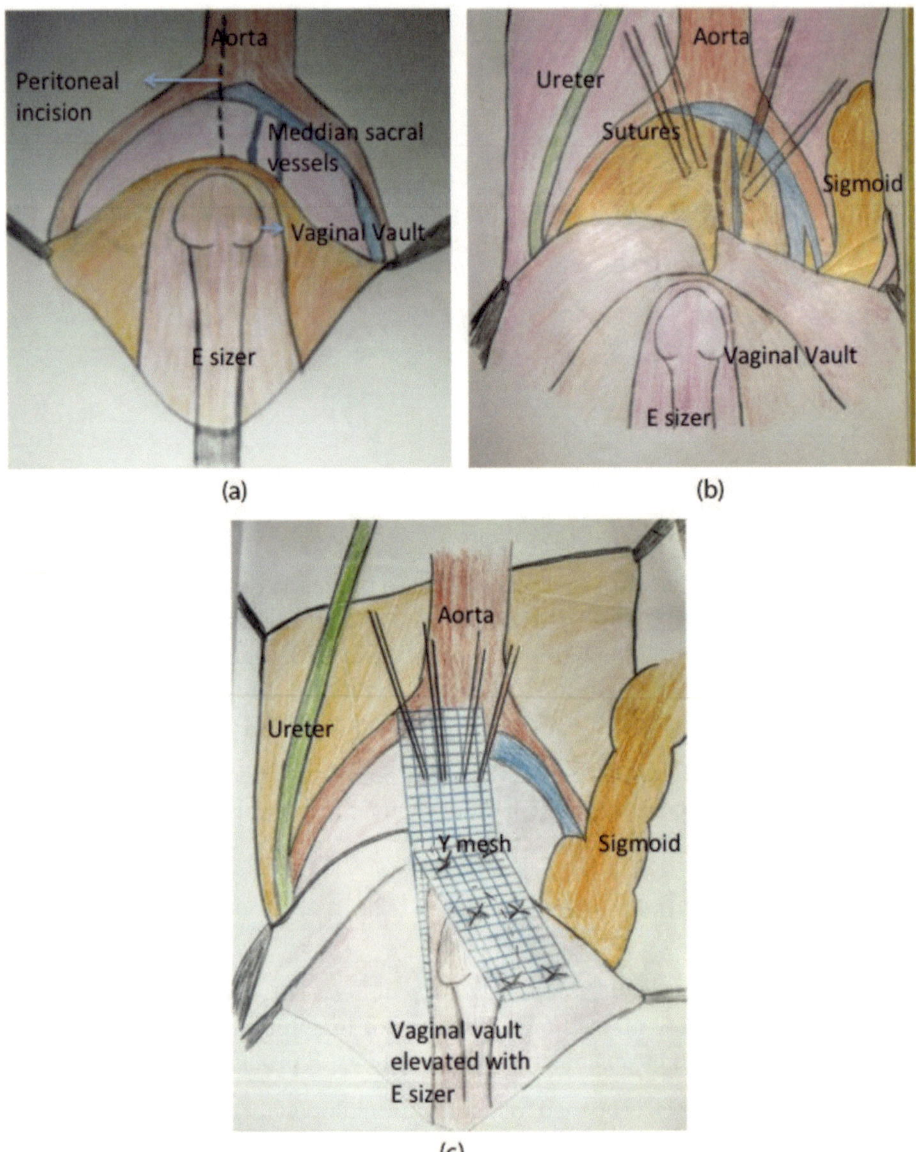

Figure 7. (a) The posterior peritoneum is incised over the sacral promontory and the median sacral artery and vein are identified. (b) Non-absorbable sutures are passed through the presacral fascia. The vaginal vault is elevated with an E-sizer and the bladder is dissected anteriorly and the rectum is dissected posteriorly. (c) The inverted oblique limbs of Y shaped mesh are anchored to the anterior and posterior vaginal wall. The vertical limb is anchored to the presacral fascia.

The vertical limb of inverted Y is now anchored to the periosteum with 2–4 nonabsorbable 0 suture. The peritoneum over the sacrum is sutured carefully taking care to prevent ureteric injury (**Figure 7(a)–(c)**). A paravaginal repair to anchor the lateral vaginal wall with arcus tendineus fascia pelvis is done. The abdomen is closed in layers. After this a posterior colporrhaphy procedure is done to correct the laxity of the perineal body.

9. Corrections of pelvic organ prolapse with mesh systems

Over the last decade, mesh augmented surgical repair is being increasingly used in pelvic organ prolapse. In 2008, the FDA issued a warning against the use of mesh for prolapse and incontinence repair. The warning was repeated in 2011, although narrowing it to vaginal mesh used for correction of pelvic organ prolapse (not for anti-incontinence procedures or when used abdominally). These warnings arose from concerns over mesh erosion through vagina, pain, infection, bleeding, dyspareunia, organ perforation and urinary problems. While many of these complications are common to all pelvic floor repairs, mesh erosion and some type of organ perforation are surely unique to mesh and trocars used for its placement [27, 28].

10. Role of minimally invasive surgery in vaginal vault prolapse

Though the operating times are still longer than vaginal surgery, multiple studies of minimally invasive surgery, including the laparoscopic colpopexy, robotic sacrocolpopexy, show shorter hospital stays and less blood loss compared to the open abdominal approach, they are therefore presumably associated with quicker recovery and less pain.

Randomized trials of Laparoscopic sacrocolpopexy versus robotic sacrocolpopexy showed no difference in anatomical prolapse or bulge symptoms 1 year after surgery, demonstrating that long-term outcomes after these two minimally invasive approaches may be similar [29].

However, robotic assisted laparoscopy is significantly more expensive, mainly because of a longer duration of surgery (265 min for robotic sacrocolpopexy versus 199 for laparoscopic sacrocolpopexy).

11. Recurrent prolapse and stress urinary incontinence

Vault prolapse and incontinence can develop simultaneously after hysterectomy. Women with prolapse who are continent have an increased risk of developing de novo stress urinary incontinence after surgical prolapse repair. Therefore addressing stress urinary incontinence at the time of surgical intervention for prolapse is an important consideration for improving the quality of life. Performing an anti-incontinence procedure at the time of prolapse repair is effective in reducing the risks of occult stress urinary incontinence postoperatively.

12. Operations for complete eversion of vagina

The management is always surgical because the prolapse has a tendency to enlarge gradually due to increased intraabdominal pressure. The vaginal prolapse also carries a rare risk of vaginal evisceration if not treated on time.

Rarely in elderly women who are not sexually active and have comorbidities the surgical removal of vagina (colpectomy) and closing of the vaginal space (colpocleisis) can be performed. These surgeries are rarely performed due to advances in anesthesia, as safe drugs for anesthesia in elderly are now available. The surgeon should also be sensitive towards the future coital activity and the underlying issues of patient self-image [30].

13. Conclusion

The assessment of recurrent pelvic floor dysfunction can be done clinically aided with imaging. The patient records of previous surgery are important. Vaginal apical prolapse surgery should always be combined with meticulous culdoplasty to correct the enterocele that is associated with vaginal prolapse.

When the previous surgery is sacrospinous ligament suspension, recurrent anterior vaginal prolapse is common as the vaginal axis gets deflected in sacrospinous fixation and the lines of force by increased intraabdominal pressure are directed across the vagina.

Each case should be individualized; keeping in mind the etiology of recurrent prolapse and surgical correction directed towards the cause. It is unclear whether the best route of surgical reconstruction for post hysterectomy vaginal apical prolapse is abdominal or vaginal. The most proper reconstructive surgery should be site specific, individualized and based on operating surgeon's expertise and experience.

Author details

Nidhi Sharma* and Sudakshina Chakrabarti

*Address all correspondence to: drbonuramkumar@yahoo.co.in

Saveetha University, Chennai, India

References

[1] Delancey JO. Anatomic aspects of vaginal eversion after hysterectomy. American Journal of Obstetrics and Gynecology. 1992;**166**:1717-1724

[2] Ren S, Xie B, Wang J, QiguoRong. Three-dimensional modeling of the pelvic floor support systems of subjects with or without pelvic organ prolapse. BioMed Research International. 2015;**2015**:845985. http://dx.doi.org/10.11

[3] De Groat WC. Neuroanatomy and neurophysiology: Innervation of the lower urinary tract. Female urology. In: Raz S, Rodriguez L, editors. 3rd ed. Vol. 3. Philadelphia, PA: WB Saunders Company; 2008. pp. 26-46

[4] Raizada V, Mittal RK. Pelvic floor anatomy and applied physiology. Gastroenterology Clinics of North America. 2008;**37**(3):493

[5] Loubeyre P, Copercini M. Patrick Petignat and Jean Bernard Dubuisson. Levator Ani muscle complex anatomic findings in nulliparous patients at thin section MR imaging with double opacification. Radiology. 2012;**262**(2):538-543

[6] Mouchel T, Mouchel F. Basic anatomic features in Pelviperineology. Pelviperineology. Dec. 2008;**27**(4):156-159

[7] Kindra A, Larson, Yousuf A, Delancey JOL. Perineal body anatomy in living women: 3D analysis using thin slice magnetic resonance imaging. American Journal of Obstetrics and Gynecology. 2010;**203**(5):494

[8] Richard S. Snell Clinical Anatomy. 9th ed. Philadelphia: Wolters Kluver, Lippincott Williams & Wilkins; 2012

[9] Gill BC, Rackley RR. Urinary Incontinence Relevant Anatomy. http://emedicine.medscape.com/article/1988009-overview

[10] Gormley EA, Lightner DJ, Burgio KL, Chai TC, Clemens JQ, CulkinDJ, Das AK, Foster HE Jr, Scarpero HM, Tessier CD, Vasavada SP, et al. Diagnosis and treatment of overactive bladder (nonneurogenic) in adults: AUA/SUFU guideline. The Journal of Urology. 2012;**188**(6 Suppl):2455-2463. DOI: 10.1016/j.juro.2012.09.079

[11] Lucas MG, Bedretdinova D, Bosch JLHR, Burkhard F, Cruz F, Nambiar AK, Nilsson CG, De Ridder DJMK, Tubaro A, Pickard RS. EAU Guidelines on Urinary Incontinence. European Association of Urology. 2014. Available from: http://www.uroweb.org/gls/pdf/20%20Urinary%20Incontinence_LR.pdf

[12] Swift S. Validation of a simplified technique for using POPQ pelvic organ prolapse quantification system. International Urogynecology Journal. 2006;**17**:615-620

[13] Bland DR, Earle BB. Use of the pelvic organ prolapse staging system of the International Continence Society, Society of Gynecological Surgeons in Perimenopausal Women. American Journal of Obstetrics and Gynecology. 1999;**181**:1324-1328

[14] Goldman HB, Wyndaele JJ, Kaplan SA, Wang JT, Ntanios F. Defining response and non-response to treatment in-patients with overactive bladder: A systematic review. Current Medical Research and Opinion. 2014;**30**(3):509-526. DOI: 10.1185/03007995.2013.860021

[15] Barber MD, Walters MD, Bump RC. Short forms of two condition-specific quality-of-life questionnaires for women with pelvic floor disorders (PFDI-20 and PFIQ-7). American Journal of Obstetrics and Gynecology. 2005;**193**:103-113

[16] Goba GK, Legesse AY, Zelelow YB, Gebreselassie MA, Rogers RG, Kenton KS, Mueller MG. Reliability and validity of the tigrigna version of the pelvic floor distress inventory-short form 20 (PFDI-20) and pelvic floor impact questionnaire-7 (PFIQ-7). International Urogynecology Journal. 2018. DOI: 10.1007/s00192-018-3583-9. [Epub ahead of print] PMID: 29536138

[17] Price N, Jackson SR, Avery K, Brookes ST, Abrams P. Development and psychometric evaluation of the ICIQ vaginal symptoms questionnaire: The ICIQ-VS. BJOG : An International Journal of Obstetrics and Gynaecology. 2006;**113**(6):700-712. PMID: 16709214

[18] Homma Y, Kakizaki H, Yamaguchi O, et al. Assessment of overactive bladder symptoms: Comparison of 3-day bladder diary and the overactive bladder symptom score. Urology. 2011;**77**:60-64

[19] Apostolidis A, Kirana PS, Chiu G, Link C, Tsiouprou M, Hatzichristou D. Gender and age differences in the perception of bother and health care seeking for lower urinary tract symptoms: Results from the hospitalised and outpatients' profile and expectations study. European Urology. 2009;**56**:937-947

[20] Irwin DE, Milsom I, Hunskaar S, et al. Population-based survey of urinary incontinence, overactive bladder, and other lower urinary tract symptoms in five countries: Results of the EPIC study. European Urology. 2006;**50**:1306-1315

[21] RCOG and BSUG Joint Guideline 2015. Green Top Guideline No 46—Post Hysterectomy Vaginal Vault Prolapse. Available from: https://www.rcog.org.uk/globalassets/documents/guidelines/gtg-46.pdf [Published: July 24, 2015]

[22] Argirović R, Likić-Ladević I, Vrzić-Petronijević S, Petronijević M, Ladević N. Application of transvaginal sacrospinous colpopexy in the treatment of pelvic organs prolapse. Vojnosanitetski Pregled. 2005;**62**(9):637-643. Serbian. PMID: 16229205

[23] Goldberg RP, Tomezsko JE, Winkler HA, Koduri S, Culligan PJ, Sand PK. Anterior or posterior sacrospinous vaginal vault suspension: Long-term anatomic and functional evaluation. Obstetrics & Gynecology. 2001;**98**(2):199-204

[24] Vaccaro C, Karram M. High uterosacral vaginal vault suspension to repair enterocele and apical prolapse. OBG Management. 2011;**23**(6):35-43

[25] Serati M, Braga A, Bogani G, Maggiore ULR, Sorice P, Ghezzi F, Salvatore S. Iliococcygeus fixation for the treatment of apical vaginal prolapse: Efficacy and safety at 5 years of follow-up. International Urogynecology Journal. 2015;**26**(7):1007-1012. DOI: 10.1007/s00192-015-2629-5

[26] NICE. Sacrocolpopexy Using Mesh for Vaginal Vault Prolapse Repair—NICE Interventional Procedure Guideline IPG283. January 2009. https://www.nice.org.uk/guidance/ipg283/chapter/1-Guidance

[27] Alan JW. FDA safety communication: UPDATE on serious complications associated with transvaginal placement of surgical mesh for pelvic organ prolapse. The Journal of Urology. 2011;**186**(6):2328-2330

[28] Jakus SM, Shapiro A, Hall CD. Biologic and synthetic graft use in pelvic surgery: A review. Obstetrical & Gynecological Survey. 2008;**63**(4):253-266

[29] Farnam RW. Robotic uterosacral vaginal vault suspension. Journal of Minimally Invasive Gynecology. 2014;**21**(6):S20-S21

[30] De Lancey JO, Morley JW. Total colpocleisis for vaginal eversion. American Journal of Obstetrics and Gynecology. 1997;**176**:1228-1235